Surrogate Markers to Assess Efficacy of Treatment in Chronic Liver Diseases

INTERNATIONAL FALK WORKSHOP

Surrogate Markers to Assess Efficacy of Treatment in Chronic Liver Diseases

EDITED BY

J. Reichen

Institut für Klinische Pharmakologie
Universität Bern
Inselspital
Murtenstr. 35
CH-3010 Bern
Switzerland

and

R. E. Poupon

Unité de Recherches Cliniques et Epidémiologiques
INSERM U 21
16, Avenue Paul-Vaillant-Couturier
F-94807 Villejuif Cedex
France

Proceedings of the International Falk Workshop held in Basel, Switzerland, October 23–24, 1995

KLUWER ACADEMIC PUBLISHERS
DORDRECHT / BOSTON / LONDON

Distributors

for the United States and Canada: Kluwer Academic Publishers, PO Box 358, Accord Station, Hingham, MA 02018-0358, USA

for all other countries: Kluwer Academic Publishers Group, Distribution Center, PO Box 322, 3300 AH Dordrecht, The Netherlands

A catalogue record for this book is available from the British Library

ISBN 0–7923–8705–8

Library of Congress Cataloging in Publication Data

Falk Symposium (1995: Basel, Switzerland)
Surrogate markers to assess efficacy of treatment in chronic liver diseases: proceedings of the International Falk Workshop held in Basel, Switzerland, October 23–24, 1995/edited by J. Reichen and R.E. Poupon.
p. cm.
Includes bibliographical references and index.
ISBN 0–7923–8705–8 (casebound: alk. paper)
1. Liver function tests — Congresses. 2. Liver — Diseases — Prognosis — Congresses. 3. Liver — Diseases — Treatment — Evaluation — Congresses. I. Reichen, J. (Jurg) II. Poupon, R. E. III. Title.
[DNLM: 1. Liver Diseases — therapy — congresses. 2 Chronic Diseases — therapy — congresses. 3. Biological Markers — congresses.
WI 700 F191s 1996
RC847. F35 1995
616.3′ 62—dc20
DNLM/DLC
for Library of Congress 96–17380
CIP

Copyright

Published in the United Kingdom by Kluwer Academic Publishers, PO Box 55, Lancaster, UK.

Kluwer Academic Publishers BV incorporates the publishing programmes of D. Reidel, Martinus Nijhoff, Dr W. Junk and MTP Press.

Typeset by EXPO Holdings, Malaysia

Printed and bound in Great Britain by Hartnolls Ltd., Bodmin, Cornwall.

Contents

SECTION V: CHRONIC LIVER DISEASES

List of Principal Authors

J.-P. Aboulker
INSERM SC10
16, avenue Paul-Vaillant-Couturier
F-94807 Villejuif Cedex
France

M. Bernardi
Istituto di Patologia Medica I
Policlinico S. Orsola
Via Massarenti 9
I-40138 Bologna
Italy

U. Beuers
Medizinische Klinik II
Klinikum Grosshadern
Marchioninistr. 15
D-81377 Munich
Germany

J. Bosch
School of Medicine
University of Barcelona
Hospital Clinic i Provincial
Villarroel 170
E-08036 Barcelona
Spain

R. A. Branch
Center for Clinical Pharmacology
University of Pittsburgh
Scaife Hall, Room 623
Pittsburgh
PA 15261
USA

E. Christensen
Department of Medicine B
Bispebjerg University Hospital
Bispebjerg Bakke 23
DK-2400 Copenhagen NV
Denmark

A. J. Chwalow
INSERM Unité 21
16, avenue Paul-Vaillant-Couturier
F-94807 Villejuif Cedex
France

H. U. Fisch
Psychiatrische Universitätspoliklinik
Murtenstr. 21
CH-3010 Bern
Switzerland

R. P. Jazrawi
St George's Hospital Medical School
Cranmer Terrace
London SW17 ORE
UK

E. Lotterer
Department of Internal Medicine I
University of Halle-Wittenberg
Ernst-Grube-Strasse 40
D-06120 Halle/Saale
Germany

N. McIntyre
University Department of Medicine
Royal Free Hospital
Pond Street
London NW3 2QG
UK

C. Merkel
Department of Clinical Medicine
University of Padua
Via Giustiniani 2
I-35128 Padova
Italy

L. Pagliaro
Istituto di Medica Generale e
Pneumologia
Clinica Medica R
Ospedele V. Cervello
ViaTrabucco 180
I-90146 Palermo
Italy

C. Peck
Georgetown University Medical Center
Room NE 403, Medical and Dental
Building
3900 Reservoir Road NW
Washington
DC 20007
USA

B. Portmann
Institute of Liver Studies
King's College Hospital
Bessemer Road
London SE5 9PJ
UK

R. E. Poupon
INSERM Unité 21
16, avenue Paul-Vaillant-Couturier
F-94807 Villejuif Cedex
France

G. Ramadori
Abteilung Gastroenterologie
Medizinische Universitätsklinik
Robert-Koch-Strasse 40
D-37075 Göttingen
Germany

J. Reichen
Institut für Klinische Pharmakologie
Universitat Bern
Inselspital
Murtenstr. 35
CH-3010 Bern
Switzerland

J. Schölmerich
Klinik und Poliklinik für Innere
Medizin I
Universität Regensburg
D-93042 Regensburg
Germany

D. Schuppan
Universitätsklinikum Steglitz
Medizinische Klinik, Innere Medizin
Hindenbergdamm 30
D-12202 Berlin
Germany

N. Tygstrup
Rigshospitalet
Med AFD A-2152
Blegdamsvej 9
DK-2100 Copenhagen
Denmark

P. W. F. Wilson
Framingham Heart Study
National Heart Lung and Blood Institute
5 Thurber Street
Framingham
MA 01701
USA

Introduction

R. E. POUPON

This book is composed of lectures and some of the posters presented at the international Falk workshop 'Surrogate markers to assess the efficacy of treatment in chronic liver diseases' held in October 1995 in Basel, Switzerland.

In chronic liver disease, as in all chronic diseases, the objectives associated with the development of new treatments are, in order of priority: to cure the disease; to slow the progression of the disease and to prolong survival; and to reduce morbidity with a minimum of adverse effects. If the objective is to evaluate the effectiveness of a new treatment on the survival of patients with a chronic disease, a therapeutic trial should be characterized by the inclusion of a very large number of patients, follow-up over a period of years and a significant number of deaths. Obviously, this situation immediately poses problems: generic ethical problems such as that of conducting long-term studies in an era where medical knowledge and progress are rapidly changing. In addition, ethical problems at the individual level include patient participation in a double-blind study over a long period of time. There are also organizational and financial constraints that make these studies difficult to manage. The major problem that confronts us is to obtain rapid results, using as endpoints those events that precede death: surrogate endpoints.

The classic definition of a surrogate endpoint is 'a substitute for a "true" endpoint in a clinical setting, that is a substitute for mortality or a clinical event'. To illustrate this with a concrete example let us take the evaluation of ursodeoxycholic acid in primary biliary cirrhosis. In this illness, as described in Chapter 18, there is no validated surrogate endpoint. We were therefore obliged to use a 'hard endpoint', i.e. liver transplantation or death. Under these conditions, demonstrating the effectiveness of ursodeoxycholic acid versus a placebo, required a four-year follow-up of approximately 150 patients, five years to form a conclusion. If we admit that ursodeoxycholic acid is currently the treatment of reference, to show the superiority of a new treatment, using the hard endpoint, a group of approximately 1000 patients, followed for an identical period would be necessary. What is obvious is that in the absence of a surrogate endpoint we have, more or less, reached an impasse.

In primary biliary cirrhosis, among the criteria that are currently available as substitutes for hard endpoints are 'soft endpoints'. A soft endpoint could be an indication of aggravation of the illness (e.g. an increase in bilirubinaemia associated with the appearance of a clinical complication), a score, even bilirubinaemia *per se*.

In order to look at the steps that permit the validation of soft endpoints as surrogate endpoints, it is useful to review the properties of a surrogate endpoint. Statistically, the surrogate must fulfil two conditions: (1) it must be correlated with the true endpoint; and (2) a therapeutic effect on the surrogate must correspond to a beneficial effect on the true endpoint. From a pathophysiological perspective, there must be a strong rational base justifying that the surrogate endpoint is directly associated with the hard endpoint. It should be stressed that the performance of the surrogate endpoint will depend on the pertinence of this rationale. In other words, it will capture a sizeable part of the information contained in the hard endpoint. The reader can find examples of surrogate endpoints that have been validated in areas other than hepatology in the first chapters of this book.

It is important to keep in mind some fallacies about the use of surrogate endpoints: (1) a correlation between a surrogate endpoint and survival time does not necessarily imply that the treatment effect on a surrogate endpoint will predict the treatment effect on survival; and (2) the surrogate endpoint may not be valid for drugs that have different mechanisms of action.

One of the major applications of surrogate markers is in therapeutic trials, where the objective is to reduce the sample size or the duration of a clinical trial, to make new trials more ethically feasible. Other applications would also be extremely useful. Surrogate markers may be used as substitutes for an invasive examination, for example, the serum markers of fibrosis could be used as surrogate endpoints for liver biopsies. In addition, other markers such as quality of life, which do not replace but complement hard endpoints, should also be considered.

I believe that this workshop has been very interesting, as much for the 'newness' of this subject within the context of the 'Basel Liver Week' as for the review of surrogate endpoints for use with different chronic liver diseases. It is unfortunate that, except for the Child–Pugh score for cirrhosis, the criteria discussed are better classified as potential rather than validated markers. We can only hope that this workshop, whose theme represented a 'first' in liver disease, will stimulate the validation of and/or research into the development of new surrogate endpoints in this field.

Section 1
General Considerations on Surrogate Markers

1
Surrogate markers in AIDS clinical trials

J.-P. ABOULKER

Human immunodeficiency virus (HIV) infection, in spite of the great advance in treatment recently reported with combination therapy[1,2], remains a life-threatening disease.

Understanding of the pathogenesis of the disease has changed with the use of potent HIV inhibitors and the introduction of quantitative assays to monitor HIV viral load in individual patients. It has been demonstrated[3–5] that the virus replicates very actively even during the asymptomatic phase of the disease, which was formerly thought to be a phase of latency of the infection. It has been estimated that half the amount of virus in peripheral blood is cleared and renewed every 1 or 2 days, leading to an average daily production of one billion viral particles.

The availability of additional licensed or experimental antiretroviral drugs and the development of assays in order to quantitate viral load, will increasingly encourage clinicians to start therapy earlier in the course of the disease, and to switch to alternative drugs as soon as the treatment fails in suppressing viral replication. This strategy of early intervention focused on viral load must, however, still take into account the primary objective of the treatment: prolonging survival and delaying clinical disease progression. Therefore, the key issue concerning the evaluation of different treatments is to determine how they improve clinical outcome. This is best achieved in phase III randomized trials with clinical endpoints.

However, studies carried out in patient populations with little or no experience of antiretroviral treatment have to be wide (over a thousand participants) because clinical events are rare during the early or intermediary stage of the disease, and long-lasting (over 2 years); this is a problem since a large proportion of the participants cannot stay on their assigned therapies for the whole duration of the trial.

Alternatively, attempts to introduce intermediate endpoints in clinical trials have mainly focused on the CD4 cell count; these have not provided convincing results to date. Two new facts might alter the situation:

- Due to the advances in antiretroviral treatment, several trials have detected considerable differences in clinical outcome between treatment groups that can be analysed in relation to the changes in biological markers.
- The measurement of viral load *in vivo* is performed in most clinical trials.

Figure 1 indicates the parameters that can be observed and measured in individual patients. AIDS defining parameters have been used as the gold standard in phase III efficiency trials for 10 years. Although they include a wide variety of clinical manifestations such as the wasting syndrome, opportunistic infections, neurological diseases (encephalopathy, peripheral neuropathy) and cancers (Kaposi's sarcoma, lymphomas), it has been shown that they strongly affect survival, even though the respective influence of the diverse AIDS events on survival is variable[6,7]. Furthermore, they impair the quality of life, because they frequently lead to severe sequelae and necessitate maintainance therapy with consequent side-effects.

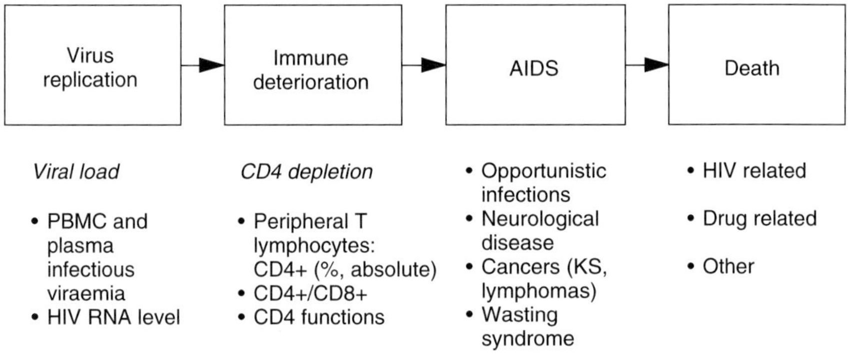

Fig. 1 HIV disease: What can be observed and measured in the patient

Of great importance for the calculation of sample size and study design, is the fact that AIDS defining events are about twice as frequent as deaths in most phase III efficacy trials[8–10], whereas death rarely occurs in non-AIDS patients. This explains why most clinical trials, designed to determine the combined endpoint of progression to AIDS or death, have not detected significant differences in survival between the treatment arms. Consequently, the validity of clinical endpoints as surrogates for death in clinical trials has not been formally established, although this might be regarded as unimportant since clinical disease progression does include both death and AIDS events.

Immune deterioration is the major landmark of HIV disease. It has qualitative and quantitative aspects. Qualitative impairment of immunity is not routinely assessed even in clinical trials because most assays remain research tools. Assays for T-lymphocyte proliferative response, HIV-specific cytolytic T-lymphocyte activity and cytokine production cannot be widely performed because they are too labour intensive. In contrast, the CD4 lymphocyte count is easy to obtain and has a central role in the follow-up of every HIV-positive individual, because most therapeutic decisions depend on the degree of immunodeficiency. It has been demonstrated to be the strongest prognostic marker of disease progression, and it has been used in almost all clinical trials to date. The effects on the CD4 cell count of antiretroviral therapy are variable. The increase is small (30–50 cells/mm^3) and of short duration (3–6 months) with nucleoside analogues such as zidovudine, didanosine, zalcitabine, lamivudine, etc., used individually. Increases of much greater magnitude (80–150 cells/mm^3) and duration (>6–12 months) have been recently reported with potent protease inhibitors and combinations of two or more drugs.

The CD4 cell count has not yet been formally validated as a surrogate marker of clinical disease progression in antiretroviral clinical trials. According to the conditions established by Prentice[11], the CD4 cell count, in order to be a valid surrogate marker, should fully represent the effect of treatment on the true endpoint of AIDS or death. This validation requires studies showing a significant treatment effect on the true endpoint of at least 3 to 4 standard deviations, and events in sufficient numbers to be statistically reliable. A state-of-the-art conference organized in June 1993 and sponsored by the US National Institute of Health reviewed the results of the 16 clinical trials available at that time, and showed that none of these trials yielded a treatment effect significant enough to allow a correct validation of the CD4 endpoint.

Furthermore, the treatment effect on CD4 cell count was not consistent with the effect on clinical outcome in several of these 16 trials. It has been shown, in monotherapy trials with nucleoside analogues, that CD4 cell count as an endpoint, even with the strongest definition of a 50% drop from baseline value which has often been used in clinical trials, cannot replace AIDS or death endpoint for assessing the treatment effect on clinical outcome. In the Concorde trial[8], which compared immediate versus deferred use of zidovudine in asymptomatic HIV infected patients, a moderate (25 to 35 cells) but highly significant difference in CD4 cell count was observed between both arms of the study throughout the three-year follow up period, leading to significant differences in time to a CD4 decline of 50% from baseline or a value of less than 200 cells. In contrast, rates of progression to AIDS or death were nearly identical in both groups, a higher (but not significant) number of deaths even being observed in the immediate group. Similar discrepancies between CD4 and clinical endpoints have been reported in other trials[12–14].

We may hope that the disappointing results obtained with the CD4 marker during monotherapy with nucleoside analogues will not be the rule with any new treatment. The Delta study, which is comparing combinations of zidovudine plus didanosine or zalcitabine to zidovudine alone, in patients with 50–350 CD4 cells, has shown a substantial treatment effect on survival, with a concomitant, marked and sustained effect on the CD4 response. Similar findings have been reported in the ACTG 175 trial which assessed the same combinations as the Delta study, and also didanosine monotherapy, in patients with CD4 cell counts between 200 and 500/mm^3.

Viral loads assays, which mainly involve the titration of infectious virus in plasma and in peripheral blood mononuclear cells and the determination of the amount of HIV RNA in plasma, have been introduced in clinical trials and observational studies during the last few years. Data are currently accumulating concerning their ability to predict clinical outcome and to replace hard clinical endpoints in the evaluation of antiretroviral therapy.

Evidence of a relationship between a high viral load and a risk of rapid clinical progression has been established in several studies[15,16], and results from large cohorts and trials should soon be available. We should learn, from frequent monitoring of both CD4 cell count and HIV RNA level in individual patients, to what extent viral replication determines immune deterioration. We may also be able to draw important conclusions from these data for the clinical and therapeutic management of HIV infected patients.

Only limited results are readily available concerning the surrogacy of viral load in clinical trials[17]. It is expected that ongoing studies in the Delta, ACTG 175 and other recently completed trails will determine to what extent improvement in clinical outcome can be predicted from therapy-induced viral load modification. Conversely, we hope to learn from these studies how much the effect of antiretroviral treatment upon viral replication must be increased in order to show a clinically significant therapeutic advance.

References

1. Yeni P for the Delta Coordinating Committee. Preliminary results of the Delta trial [oral presentation]. Fifth European Conference on Clinical Aspects and Treatment of HIV Infection; 1995 Sept 26–29; Copenhagen, Denmark.
2. Hammer S, Katzenstein D, Hughes M, Gundacker H, Hirsch M, Merigan T for the ACTG 175 Study team. Nucleoside monotherapy versus combination therapy in HIV-infected adults: a randomized, double-blind, placebo-controlled trial in persons with CD4 cell counts 200–500/mm^3. *35th International Conference on Antimicrobial Chemo therapy*. San Francisco, USA, September 1995 [Abstract LB1].
3. Coffin JM. HIV population dynamics *in vivo*: Implications for genetic variation, pathogenesis, and therapy. Science. 1995;267:483–9.
4. Ho DD, Neumann AV, Perelson AS, Chen W, Leonard JM, Markowitz M. Rapid turnover of plasma virions and CD4 lymphocytes in HIV infection. Nature. 1995;373:123–6.
5. Wei X, Ghosh SK, Taylor ME *et al.* Viral dynamics in human immunodeficiency virus type 1 infection. Nature. 1995;373:117–22.
6. Oksenhendler E, Charreau I, Tournerie C. *Toxoplasma gondii* infection in advanced HIV infection. AIDS. 1994;8:483–7.
7. Neaton JD, Wentworth DN, Rhame F, Hogan C, Abrams DI, Deyton L. Methods of studying interventions – Considerations in choice of a clinical endpoint for AIDS clinical trials. Stat in Med. 1994;13:2107–25.
8. Concorde Coordinating Committee. CONCORDE:MRC/ANRS randomised double-blind controlled trial of immediate and deferred zidovudine in symptom-free HIV infection. Lancet. 1994;343: 871–81.
9. Kahn JO, Lagakos SW, Richman DD *et al.* A controlled trial comparing zidovudine with didanosine in human immunodeficiency virus infection. N Engl J Med. 1992;327:581–7.
10. Fischl MA, Stanley K, Collier AC *et al.* Combination and monotherapy with Zidovudine and Zalcitabine in patients with advanced HIV disease. Ann Intern Med. 1995;122:24–32.
11. Prentice RL. Surrogate endpoints in clinical trials: definition and operational criteria. Stat in Med. 1989;8:431–40.
12. Abrams DI, Goldman A, Launer C *et al.* A comparative trial of didanosine and zalcitabine in patients with human immunodeficiency virus infection who are intolerant of or have failed zidovudine therapy. N Engl J Med. 1994;330:657–62.
13. Darbyshire JH, Aboulker JP. Didanosine for zidovudine-intolerant patients with HIV disease (Letter to the Editor). Lancet. 1992;1346–7.
14. Volberding PA, Lagakos SW, Grimes JM *et al.* for the AIDS clinical trials group. A comparison of immediate with deferred zidovudine therapy for asymptomatic HIV-infected adults with CD4 cell counts of 500 or more per cubic millimeter. N Engl J Med. 1995;333:401–7.

15. Mellors JW, Kingsley LA, Rinaldo CR *et al.* Quantitation of HIV-1 RNA plasma predicts outcome after seroconversion. Ann Intern Med. 1995;122:573–9.
16. Saksela K, Stevens C, Rubinstein P, Baltimore D. Human immunodeficiency virus type 1 mRNA expression in peripheral blood cells predicts disease progression independently of the numbers of CD4+ lymphocytes. Proc Natl Acad Sci USA. 1994;91:1104–8.
17. Crumpacker C, Nelles S, Yen-Lieberman B *et al.* Correlation of plasma HIV-1 RNA level and development of resistance mutations to AZT and DDI with disease progression in patients with advanced HIV-1 disease and little or no AZT therapy. Abstract 42. Fourth International Workshop on HIV drug resistance; 1995 July 6–9; Sardinia, Italy.

2
Surrogate markers and prediction of cardiovascular disease

P. W. F. WILSON

LOGISTIC REGRESSION AND PREDICTION EQUATIONS

Coronary disease prediction rests on the principle of measuring several factors, following a population, and relating baseline values to clinical or subclinical outcomes. The simplest form taken is a 2×2 table, where a screening test is either positive or negative and the outcome, or event, is likewise positive or negative. The first extension of prediction is the $2 \times n$ table, where there are n possibilities for the test variable and again only a positive or negative outcome. It is then possible to test for a significant relationship across the n test strata and the outcome using the chi-square test.

Large scale population based investigations such as the Framingham Heart Study, were undertaken in the late 1940s to study the relation between a variety of factors and the occurrence of cardiovascular diseases (CVD). Early reports from Framingham showed that age, cholesterol level, blood pressure (either systolic or diastolic) and cigarette smoking were each related to the occurrence of coronary heart disease (CHD)[1]. It was readily appreciated that the chi-square approach had its limitations, as the analysis considered only one factor at a time. For instance, the relation CHD and several levels of cholesterol and CHD could be tested with the $2 \times n$ chi-square approach mentioned above. Proceeding further with the analysis, the investigator could stratify the data by a second independent variable, such as age categories, and perform separate analyses for cholesterol levels and CHD for each of the age strata.

Although only a few variables, such as sex, age, cholesterol, blood pressure, smoking and diabetes, were available in the 1950s, the number of separate calculations to test for associations with CHD was very large. Technology was also a limiting factor, as statisticians typically only had IBM card sorters and mechanical calculators at their disposal. Once stratification by second, or possibly third, level variables was undertaken, the number of calculations became extremely large. An advantage of this approach was knowledge of the actual number of persons at risk in the various strata. Where data were particularly sparse for various combinations of variables, it became evident that estimates of CHD risk for these subsets were relatively unreliable.

A novel statistical technique was developed to deal with the relation of multiple factors to CHD in the 1960s. It employed regression methods, available in the past to predict continuous variables using linear models, and adapted these techniques to the prediction of dichotomous (yes/no) events. The logit function was used in the calculations and the technique was named logistic regression[2]. In its earliest adaptations, variables such as age, cholesterol, blood pressure and systolic pressure were used to predict CHD over a fixed time interval. As the relations between the variables and CHD differed for men and women, separate analyses were performed for each sex. Many person-hours of mechanical calculations were required to accomplish this task. Early Framingham requisition slips show purchase orders 'to invert a variance–covariance matrix as required for a logistic regression analysis' for the solution of these problems.

The product of logistic regression was an equation that best fitted the data for test factors (independent variables) and outcome (dependent variable). An example of such a formulation is shown below. The dependent variable is CHD and the probability of its occurrence is represented as a quotient. The key components of this equation are the individual beta (β) coefficients and their associated variables[2,3]. The standard error for each of the beta estimates is used to calculate 95% confidence intervals for the estimates.

$$\text{Prob}_{\text{CHD}} = \frac{1}{1 + e^{-\{\beta_0 + \beta_1 (\text{age}) + \beta_2 (\text{cholesterol}) + \beta_3 (\text{systolic pressure}) + \beta_4 (\text{smoking}) + \beta_5 (\text{HDL-C})\}}} . \quad [1]$$

As an illustration, in the equation above, the β_0 term represents the intercept, β_1 is the coefficient for age, β_2 is the coefficient for cholesterol, β_3 is the coefficient for systolic blood pressure, β_4 is the coefficient for cigarette smoking within the past year, and β_5 is the coefficient for HDL cholesterol.

The relation between a specific variable and the outcome can be shown by multiplying the coefficient by the number of units of interest for the variable, and exponentiating this product, as shown in Table 1 for a sample analysis, based on an earlier report of CHD prevalence in the Framingham Offspring sample. The columns give the factors, beta coefficients and the standard error of

Table 1 Multivariate logistic regression coefficients and relative odds for prevalent CHD (Framingham Offspring 1971)

Factor	*Beta coefficient*	*Standard deviation beta*	*Unit*	*Relative odds*	*95% CI of relative odds*
Constant β_0)	9.65	2.06			
Age (β_1)	0.1221	0.0340	10 years	3.39	1.74–6.60
Cholesterol (β_2)	0.0106	0.0036	10 mg/dl (0.26 mmol/L)	1.11	1.04–1.19
Systolic pressure (β_3)	–0.0008	0.0010	10 mm Hg	1.00	0.97–1.01
Smoking (β_4)	0.1580	0.3334	1 (yes/no)	1.17	0.61–2.25
HDL-C (β_5)	–0.0400	0.0165	5 mg/dl (0.13 mmol/L)	0.82	0.70–0.96

the beta coefficients. As shown below, multiplying the beta coefficient by the unit measure of interest and then exponentiating the result gives an estimate of the relative odds associated with a unit difference in the factor considered.

$$\text{Relative odds}_{\text{estimate}} = e^{(\beta_i \times \text{unit})} \quad [2]$$
$$\text{Relative odds}_{\text{lower 95\% CI}} = e^{(\beta_i - 1.96 \times SD\beta_i) \times \text{unit}} \quad [3]$$
$$\text{Relative odds}_{\text{upper 95\% CI}} = e^{(\beta_i + 1.96 \times SD\beta_i) \times \text{unit}} \quad [4]$$

For instance, calculation of the relative odds associated with total cholesterol and CHD prevalence in the Framingham Offspring in 1971[4], would be $e^{(0.0106 \times 10)}$ or $e^{(0.106)} = 1.11$. From equation [3], the lower confidence interval of the relative odds estimate is $e^{\{(0.0106 - 1.96\,(0.0036)\} \times 10} = 1.04$, and from [4] the upper confidence interval of the relative odds estimate is 1.19.

PRACTICAL APPLICATION OF LOGISTIC MODELS

The researcher should carefully consider the variables used to predict an outcome. Testing specific hypotheses is preferred and candidate variables should be proposed before calculations are performed. Many investigators frown upon the use of stepwise regression techniques in CHD prediction as such an approach typically indicates that a formal null hypothesis was not developed prior to undertaking the analysis. For example, an investigator may be interested in whether obesity is related to the occurrence of heart disease. It would be appropriate to test whether age and an obesity measure (for example body mass index or relative weight) are significantly associated with CHD. Age is almost always included in CHD prediction analyses as it is highly associated with the outcome, and the initial research question is typically whether a given factor is important over and above age. An expected result would be increased relative odds for CHD associated with both age and obesity.

Typical uses of logistic regression require 50 or more cases, usually at least several hundred controls, and a small set of independent variables that are potentially related to the outcome. The estimates are most reliable for those which are relatively typical of the populations. As taken from Table 1[4], factors associated with the prevalence of CHD in the Framingham Offspring sample were estimated for men (39 cases, 1250 controls) between the ages of 35–54 years; cholesterol, systolic blood pressure, smoking and HDL-C were considered. Most persons with CHD had mild elevations in one, two or three of these factors. It is unreasonable to try to estimate the CHD risk for an individual with extreme values of all four of these variables, as there are relatively few people with such a risk factor profile and the predictions are largely extrapolations of the data[5–7].

Multivariate logistic regression can also be incidence data, and in this case it is preferable to use time dependent formulations, such as the Cox model[8]. Such approaches have been used in the Framingham Study to estimate CHD and stroke incidence over time. Taking the beta coefficients, simple score sheets were developed to aid practitioners in the assessment of CHD risk (Table 2) and stroke risk (Table 3)[9,10]. An example of the their application to a typical Framingham participant at risk for heart disease is shown in Figure 1. Logistic

Table 2 Coronary heart disease risk factor prediction chart

1. Find points for each risk factor

Age (if female)				*Age (if male)*				*HDL cholesterol*		*Cholesterol*		*Systolic BP*			
Age	*Pts*	*Age*	*Pts*	*Age*	*Pts*	*Age*	*Pts*	*HDL-C*	*Pts*	*Total-C*	*Pts*	*SBP*	*Pts*	*Other*	*Pts*
30	–12	47–48	5	30	–2	57–59	13	25–26	7	139–151	–3	98–104	–2	Cigarettes	4
31	–11	49–50	6	31	–1	60–61	14	27–29	6	152–166	–2	105–112	–1	Diabetic – male	3
32	–9	51–52	7	32–33	0	62–64	15	30–32	5	167–182	–1	113–120	0	Diabetic – female	6
33	–8	53–55	8	34	1	65–67	16	33–35	4	183–199	0	121–129	1	ECG-LVH	9
34	–6	56–60	9	35–36	2	68–70	17	36–38	3	200–219	1	130–139	2		
35	–5	61–67	10	37–38	3	71–73	18	39–42	2	220–239	2	140–149	3	0 pts for each No	
36	–4	68–74	11	39	4	74	19	43–46	1	240–262	3	150–160	4		
37	–3			40–41	5			47–50	0	263–288	4	161–172	5		
38	–2			42–43	6			51–55	–1	289–315	5	173–185	6		
39	–1			44–45	7			56–60	–2	316–330	6				
40	0			46–47	8			61–66	–3						
41	1			48–49	9			67–73	–4						
42–43	2			50–51	10			74–80	–5						
44	3			52–54	11			81–87	–6						
45–56	4			55–56	12			88–96	–7						

2. Sum points for all risk factors

_____ + _____ + _____ + _____ + _____ + _____ + _____ = _____
Age HDL–C Total–C SBP Smoker Diabetes ECG–LVH Point total

Note: Minus points substract from total

Table 2 Continued

3. Look up risk corresponding to point total												4. Compare to average 10-year risk		
	Probability			*Probability*			*Probability*			*Probability*			*Probability*	
Pts	*5 Yr*	*10 Yr*	*Pts*	*5 Yr*	*10 Yr*	*Pts*	*5 Yr*	*10 Yr*	*Pts*	*5 Yr*	*10 Yr*	*Age*	*Women*	*Men*
≤1	<1%	<2%	10	2%	6%	19	8%	16%	28	19%	33%	30–34	<1%	3%
2	1%	2%	11	3%	6%	20	8%	18%	29	20%	36%	35–39	<1%	5%
3	1%	2%	12	3%	7%	21	9%	19%	30	22%	38%	40–44	2%	6%
4	1%	2%	13	3%	8%	22	11%	21%	31	24%	40%	45–49	5%	10%
5	1%	3%	14	4%	9%	23	12%	23%	32	25%	42%	50–54	8%	14%
6	1%	3%	15	5%	10%	24	13%	25%				55 59	12%	16%
7	1%	4%	16	5%	12%	25	14%	27%				60–64	13%	21%
8	2%	4%	17	6%	13%	26	16%	29%				65–69	9%	30%
9	2%	5%	18	7%	14%	27	17%	31%				70–74	12%	24%

After Anderson[9]

Table 3 Stroke risk factor prediction chart

1. Find points for each risk factor

Men (pts)								*Women (pts)*							
Age	*BP (mm Hg)*	*HYP Rx*	*Diabetes*	*Cigs*	*CVD*	*AF*	*LVH*	*Age*	*SBP*	*HYP Rx*	*Diabetes*	*Cigs*	*CVD*	*AF*	*LVH*
54–56 = 0	95–105 = 0	No = 0	No = 0	No = 0	No = 0	No = 0	No = 0	54–56 = 0	95–104 = 0	No = 0	No = 0	No = 0	No = 0	No = 0	No = 0
57–59 = 1	106–116 = 1	Yes = 2	Yes = 2	Yes = 2	Yes = 4	Yes = 4	Yes = 6	57–59 = 1	105–114 = 1	If Yes	Yes = 3	Yes = 3	Yes = 2	Yes = 6	Yes = 4
60–62 = 2	117–126 = 2							60–62 = 2	115–124 = 2	see					
63–65 = 3	127–137 = 3							63–65 = 3	125–134 = 3	below					
66–68 = 4	138–148 = 4							66–68 = 4	135–144 = 4						
69–71 = 5	149–159 = 5							69–71 = 5	145–154 = 5						
72–74 = 6	160–170 = 6							72–74 = 6	155–164 = 6						
75–77 = 7	171–181 = 7							75–77 = 7	165–174 = 7						
78–80 = 8	182–191 = 8							78–80 = 8	175–184 = 8						
81–83 = 9	192–202 = 9							81–83 = 9	185–194 = 9						
84–86 = 10	203–213 = 10							84–86 = 10	195–204 = 10						

If currently under antihypertensive therapy add the following points depending on SBP level

SBP	95–104	105–114	115–124	125–134	
Pts	(6)	(5)	(5)	(4)	
SBP	135–144	145–154			
Pts	(3)	(3)			
SBP	155–164	165–174	175–184	185–194	195–204
Pts	(2)	(1)	(1)	(0)	(0)

2. Sums points for all risk factors

_____ + _____ + _____ + _____ + _____ + _____ + _____ + _____ = _____

Age + HDL-C + HYP Rx + Diabetes + Cigs + CVD + AF + LVH = Point total

Note: Minus points substract from total

Table 3 Continued

3. Look up risk corresponding to point total												4. Compare to average 10-year risk			
Men 10-year probability						*Women 10-year probability*						*Avg 10-year prob by age*			
Pts	*Prob*	*Pts*	*Prob*	*Pts*	*Prob*	*Pts*	*Prob*	*Pts*	*Prob*	*Pts*	*Prob*	*Men*		*Women*	
1	2.6%	11	11.2%	21	41.7%	1	1.1%	11	7.6%	21	43.4%	55–59	5.9%	55–59	3.0%
2	3.0%	12	12.9%	22	46.6%	2	1.3%	12	9.2%	22	50.0%	60–64	7.8%	60–64	4.7%
3	3.5%	13	14.8%	23	51.8%	3	1.6%	13	11.1%	23	57.0%	65–69	11.0%	65–69	7.2%
4	4.0%	14	17.0%	24	57.3%	4	2.0%	14	13.3%	24	64.2%	70–74	13.7%	70–74	10.9%
5	4.7%	15	19.5%	25	62.8%	5	2.4%	15	16.0%	25	71.4%	75–79	18.0%	75–79	15.5%
6	5.4%	16	22.4%	26	68.4%	6	2.9%	16	19.1%	26	78.2%	80–84	22.3%	80–84	23.9%
7	6.3%	17	25.5%	27	73.8%	7	3.5%	17	22.8%	27	84.4%				
8	7.3%	18	29.0%	28	79.0%	8	4.3%	18	27.0%						
9	8.4%	19	32.9%	29	83.7%	9	5.2%	19	31.9%						
10	9.7%	20	37.1%	30	87.9%	10	6.3%	20	37.3%						

Keys for symbols

SBP – Systolic blood pressure
HYP Rx – Under antihypertensive therapy?
Diabetes – History of diabetes?
Cigs – Smokes cigarettes?
From Wolf[10]

CVD – History of myocardial infarction, angina pectoris, coronary insufficiency, intermittent claudication or congestive heart failure?
AV – History of atrial fibrillation?
LVH – Left ventricular hypertrophy on ECG?

regression techniques test for statistical associations and such associations are not necessarily causative. The typical criteria for causation are that an association with an outcome be strong, graded, independent of other effects, consistent across studies, reversible with a therapy or intervention, and biologically plausible.

Generalizability of prediction equations cannot always be assumed. For instance, CHD prediction in middle class American Caucasians may not necessarily hold for other ethnic groups, different age groups, and persons with underlying conditions, such as pre-existing heart disease. Often the equations can be used to categorize, or rank, persons from other groups, but absolute levels of risk may not be accurate. Framingham CHD equations have been applied to population studies from Honolulu and Israel. In each case the relative rank for CHD risk, but the not the absolute risk, was thought to be well estimated[11].

OTHER INVESTIGATIVE ISSUES

The investigator should also consider various issues that are associated with the accuracy of CHD prediction. Several factors concern the specific laboratory tests used for screening. What is the biological variability for the given test, and what is the analytical variation associated with the test in the laboratory? Often these items are overlooked. Imprecision and inaccuracy at this level can seriously hamper predictive capability. For instance, the biological variability of the total cholesterol measurement over the course of a year is approximately 6%, and the analytical variability is 3–4%[12,13]. Sampling when subjects are known to have increased variability in their measurements, such as following a recent weight change or alterations in health status, may seriously reduce the predictive potential of a test.

Multiple measures help to reduce the variability for various tests. While population studies often show a relation between a single measurement and a later outcome, often such an approach is inadequate for patient care. A single measurement may be statistically associated with an outcome, and more than one measurement may improve prediction, a phenomenon called the *regression dilution effect*[14]. On the other hand, often a study is based upon identifying a group of subjects with extreme values (either high or low) and then including them in a subsequent follow-up study with multiple observations or an intervention. In this case, if the initial value is extreme, the second value is more likely to lie closer to the population mean for that variable. As an example, if persons with cholesterol levels >300 mg/dl (7.94 mmol/L) were initially screened for a study and on follow-up the same persons had a lower value, the investigator would need to consider that some of the difference between the first and second measurements could be ascribed to *regression to the mean*. This issue is important during follow-up as regression to the mean may partly explain the ‘improvement’ in the factor under study.

SURROGATE MARKERS FOR CARDIOVASCULAR DISEASE

A variety of surrogate markers for heart disease have been proposed, including carotid artery evaluation, electrocardiogram and echocardiogram, and ankle/arm blood pressure ratios. Each is potentially a subclinical marker of atherosclerosis or physiological derangement. At another level are factors such as early manifestations of clinical disease, for example, a positive history for claudication or angina pectoris in persons who have not sought medical advice, as well as exercise, pulse rate and other items which are more often classified as primary risk factor variables.

Left ventricular hypertrophy on the electrocardiogram (ECG-LVH) has been recognized as an important risk factor for cardiovascular disease[15,16]. As an example, the odds of experiencing CVD among Framingham participants was approximately 1.5 times greater among individuals with ECG-LVH compared to those without the finding[16]. More recently, echocardiograms have been performed and left ventricular mass (LV mass) has been estimated for participants. An increase in LV mass has also been associated with subsequent CHD and stroke[17,18].

Another non-invasive surrogate measure of vascular disease that has achieved some popularity is the ankle/arm blood pressure index. A typical ratio of the systolic pressure in the arm (brachial artery) to that in the leg is 1.0 when measurements are made in supine subjects, and investigators have shown that a lower index (ankle/arm index <0.9) is associated with a greater risk of cardiovascular disease in the Cardiovascular Health Study[19].

Carotid arteries are often involved with atherosclerotic plaques, and stenosis is a marker for an increased risk of cerebrovascular disease and for generalized atherosclerosis[20]. Auscultation of a carotid bruit in the neck has been associated with a greater risk of stroke and myocardial infarction in women (approximately a threefold risk), and a lesser impact of bruit was observed for men[21]. More recent B mode ultrasound evaluations at the carotid bifurcation have graded intima–media thickness and have categorized the degree of stenosis. A multitude of cardiovascular risk factors such as smoking, hypercholesterolaemia, insulin levels, homnocysteine and elevated fibrinogen levels have been linked to abnormalities in one or both of these measures[22–26]. One investigation has tried to summarize the status of subclinical markers by taking inventory of the degree of known sublinical disease and relating its presence to subsequent risk of CHD, myocardial infarction and all cause mortality[19]. This recent report concerned approximately 5000 elderly participants in the Cardiovascular Health Study who were followed for 2.4 years in a multicentre study of persons >65 years. Persons with subclinical disease (abnormal ankle/arm index, abnormal common or internal carotid ultrasound examination, major ECG abnormalities, abnormal ejection fraction or ejection fraction on echocardiogram, questionnaires for angina pectoris or claudication) ran approximately twice the risk of subsequent clinical coronary heart disease, even after adjustment for traditional cardiovascular risk factors.

SUMMARY

The pathological sequence for persons free of disease and progression to risk factors, subclinical disease, clinical disease and death is complex. Transitions from one phase to the next occur insidiously, and strict attention needs to be paid to data collection, accurate formulation of the specific processes to be studied, and careful interpretation of the results. Choice of prediction variables is often a key item and it is especially helpful if they can be measured with accuracy and precision. Surrogate measures and study of subclinical disease offers new opportunities to study the pathological processes prior to the occurrence of clinical disease, with the hope that interventions can be studied with greater detail and hopefully lead to greater efficacy.

References

1. Dawber, TR, Moore FEJ, Mann GV. Coronary heart disease in the Framingham Study. Am J Pub Health. 1957;47:pt 2:4–24.
2. Walker SH, Duncan DB. Estimation of the probability of an event as a function of several independent variables. Biometrika. 1967;54:167–79.
3. Schlesselmann JJ. Case-control studies. New York: Oxford, 1982.
4. Garrison RJ, Wilson PWF, Feinleib M, Kannel WB, McNamara PM. Obesity and lipoprotein cholesterol in the Framingham Offspring Study. Metabolism. 1980;29:1053–60.
5. Wilson PWF, Evans JC. Coronary artery prediction. Am J Hypertens. 1993;6:309S–11S.
6. Wilson PWF, Castelli WP, Kannel WB. Coronary risk prediction in adults: The Framingham Heart Study. Am J Cardiol. 1987;59(G):91–4.
7. Wilson PWF. Total cardiovascular risk. In: Izzo JL, Black HR, editors. Hypertension primer: The essentials of high blood pressure. Dallas: American Heart Association. 1993:190–1.
8. Cox DR. Regression models and life tables. J R Stat Soc (B). 1992;34:187–220.
9. Anderson, KM, Wilson PWF, Odell PM, Kannel WB. An updated coronary risk profile. A statement for health professionals. Circulation. 1991;83:357–63.
10. Wolf, PA, D'Agostino RB, Belanger AJ, Kannel WB. Probability of stroke: A risk profile from the Framingham Study. Stroke. 1991;3:312–8.
11. Gordon T, Garcia-Palmieri MR, Kagan A, Kannel WB, Schiffman J. Differences in coronary heart disease in Framingham, Honolulu and Puerto Rico. J Chron Dis. 1974;27:329–44.
12. Cooper GR, Smith SJ, Myers GL, Sampson EJ, Magid E. Estimating and minimizing effects of biologic sources of variation by relative range when measuring the mean of serum lipids and lipoproteins. Clin Chem. 1994;40:227–32.
13. Cooper GR, Myers GL, Smith J, Schlant RC. Blood lipid measurements: Variations and practical utility. JAMA. 1992;267:1652–60.
14. MacMahon S, Peto R, Cutler J *et al.* Blood pressure, stroke, and coronary heart disease, I: Prolonged differences in blood pressure: prospective observational studies corrected for the regression dilution bias. Lancet. 1990;335:765–74.
15. Kannel WB, Dannenberg AL, Levy D. Population implications of left ventricular hypertrophy. Am J Cardiol. 1987;60:851–931.
16. Kannel WB. Left ventricular hypertrophy as a risk factor. The Framingham experience. J Hypertens. Suppl 1991;9(2):S3–8.
17. Levy D, Garrison RJ, Savage DD, Kannel WB, Castelli WP. Left ventricular mass and incidence of coronary heart disease in an elderly cohort. The Framingham Heart Study. Ann Intern Med. 1989;11:101–7.
18. Levy D, Garrison RJ, Savage DD, Kannel WB, Castelli WP. Prognostic implications of echocardiographically determined left ventricular mass in the Framingham Heart Study. N Engl J Med. 1990;322:1561–6.
19. Kuller LH, Shemanski L, Psaty BM *et al.* Subclinical disease as an independent risk factor for cardiovascular disease. Circulation. 1995;92:720–6.
20. Sutton-Tyrrell K, Alcorn HG, Herzog H, Kelsey SF, Kuller LH. Morbidity, mortality, and antihypertensive treatment effects by extent of atherosclerosis in older adults with isolated systolic hypertension. Stroke. 1995;26:1319–24.
21. Wolf PA, Kannel WB, Sorlie P, McNamara PM. Asymptomatic carotid bruit and risk of stroke. The Framingham Study. JAMA. 1981;245:1442–5.
22. Wendelhag I, Wiklund O, Wikstrand J. Arterial wall thickness in familial hypercholesterolemia. Ultrasound measurement of intima–media thickness in the common carotid artery. Arterioscler Thromb. 1992;12:70–7.

23. Tell GS, Polak JF, Ward BJ, Kittner SJ, Savage PJ, Robbins J. The Cardiovascular Health Study (CHS) Collaborative Research Group. Relation of smoking with carotid artery wall thickness and stenosis in older adults. The Cardiovascular Health Study. Circulation. 1994;90:2905–8.
24. Agewall S, Fagerberg B, Attvall S, Wendelhag I, Urbanavicius V, Wikstrand J. Carotid artery wall intima–media thickness is associated with insulin-mediated glucose disposal in men at high and low coronary risk. Stroke. 1995;26:956–60.
25. Salomaa V, Riley W, Kark JD, Nardo C, Folsom AR. Non-insulin-dependent diabetes mellitus and fasting glucose and insulin concentrations are associated with arterial stiffness indexes. The Atherosclerosis Risk in Communities Study. Circulation. 1995;91:1432–43.
26. Selhub J, Jacques PF, Bostom AG *et al.* Association between plasma homocysteine and extracranial carotid stenosis. N Engl J Med. 1995;332:286–91.

3
Requirements for surrogate markers as seen by regulatory agencies

C. PECK

Regulatory agencies such as the US FDA, have long used surrogate endpoints for approval of new drugs. Examples include blood pressure reduction as a surrogate endpoint for hypertension related stroke, heart failure, and survival; reduced ventricular premature beats (VPBs) for cardiac arrhythmia related sudden death; lowered serum cholesterol levels for coronary artery disease related morbid events; bone density and total body calcium for osteoporosis related bone fractures; increased blood proteinase inhibitor levels for alpha-1 proteinase inhibitor deficiency linked pulmonary function and emphysema; and blood CD4 cell concentrations for survival and progress of AIDS.

However, surrogate endpoints have not always been successfully correlated with clinical outcomes, as exemplified by the failure of VPBs to predict the outcome of the CAST trial. Hence the FDA has become increasingly cautious in its use of surrogate endpoints for approval of new drugs.

Regulatory scientists have cited the following principles as important considerations regarding relevance of surrogate endpoints in drug development and approval:

1. Biological plausibility.
2. Positive association between a drug effect on the surrogate endpoint and the clinical outcome.
3. Severity of the disease.
4. Availability of other therapy.
5. Toxicity of the subject drug.
6. Feasibility of conducting clinical trials with clinically meaningful endpoints.
7. Existence of ongoing studies to assess efficacy based on clinical endpoints.

Section II
Scores and Quantitative Tests

4
Quantitative liver function tests

N. TYGSTRUP

WHY QUANTIFY LIVER FUNCTION?

Patients seek medical advice for one reason: in the hope of averting the consequences of disease. The first step is to identify the disease by diagnostic procedures, but the decisive step is to estimate the consequences, i.e. the prognosis in a broad sense, and in particular whether the prognosis can be improved by treatment.

For most liver diseases the diagnosis does not *per se* indicate a precise prognosis, except perhaps in the case of hepatocellular carcinoma. The consequences of acute and chronic hepatitis and of cirrhosis vary from minor to fatal, depending on the degree of liver dysfunction. This necessitates measurement of liver function.

In many diseases, laboratory observations, which reflect the physiological role of the organ in question, will reveal the degree of dysfunction and changes resulting from treatment. However, the physiological role of the liver cannot similarly be defined by one or a few functions indispensable for health and survival. The liver is considered to be the organ which can express the greatest number of the genes in the genome, resulting in the ability to perform an estimated 5000 functions. Whether failure of one or a combination of these, or failure of as yet unknown functions, is responsible for liver failure, remains unknown.

The quantitative tests currently available are surrogates for these vital functions. The tests may be evaluated as indicators of severity by comparing them with other measures of severity, and as indicators of prognosis by clinical studies.

SURROGATES FOR SEVERITY

In the absence of a gold standard against which tests can be evaluated, their potential usefulness as a measure of the functional integrity of the liver may be estimated by their agreement with general criteria for quantitative function tests, and by comparison with other tests.

Criteria

Physiological importance

The hepatic metabolism of carbohydrate, fat and amino acids is considered to be a pivotal liver function. These metabolic processes are highly regulated by hormones, cytokines, flow and metabolic status. Tests measuring these require control of regulating factors.

Of the liver functions eliminating compounds from the blood, the drug metabolizing microsomal P450 system is considered important. It lends itself to measurement by tolerance tests, and several tests have been suggested. Focusing on this aspect of liver function is in agreement with the view that liver failure is an 'intoxication', and that the state of the microsomal detoxification system is pivotal. It is a very complex system, subject to genetic polymorphism and induction or suppression by numerous factors[1], accounting for great inter- and intra-individual variability. Figure 1 shows the fluctuation of antipyrine clearance in control subjects followed at regular intervals during a period of 3 years.

It is known that biliary obstruction may occur without liver failure. Therefore quantitative tests based on biliary excretion of a compound may not be a useful surrogate for liver function.

Kinetics

The function of most organs responds to the immediate needs of the body. This applies to liver functions which appear to be highly regulated. A damaged liver

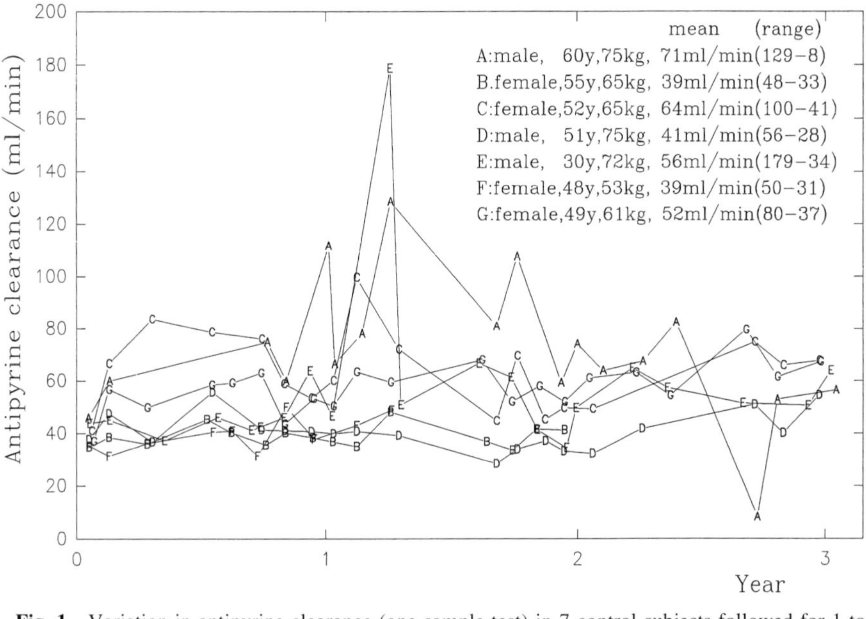

Fig. 1 Variation in antipyrine clearance (one-sample test) in 7 control subjects followed for 1 to 3 years

may perform to satisfaction as long as the demands for the function are below a certain threshold. A defect is revealed by the inability to increase the function to the level which can be obtained by the healthy liver. It is only observable as a reduction in the maximum the organ can perform when challenged, i.e. by measuring the capacity of the function. Spontaneous blood levels of physiological compounds, as with serum creatinine in kidney disease, are not reliable, being a function of production rate, elimination rate and volume of distribution. For this reason most quantitative liver tests are tolerance tests.

Correlations

Covariation between two tests indicates that they have a common determinant which can be designated 'the functional liver mass'. The concept is closely linked to 'the intact cell hypothesis' which assumes a relation between function and total hepatocyte volume. It has been supported in partially hepatectomized[2] and cirrhotic rats[3], and in patients with cirrhosis[4]. A great number of statistically significant correlations have been found, typically with correlation coefficients between 0.6 and 0.8. The common determinant (r^2), assumed to be the 'functional liver mass', thus may account for only half of the variation of the tests. The limits of the correlation are best seen with large numbers of measurements (Figure 2), because it shows that aberrant values are frequent. It becomes obvious that the tests are not equivalent.

The remaining variation must have other causes, such as analytical error, failure to measure the true capacity, influence of regulating factors; or it could

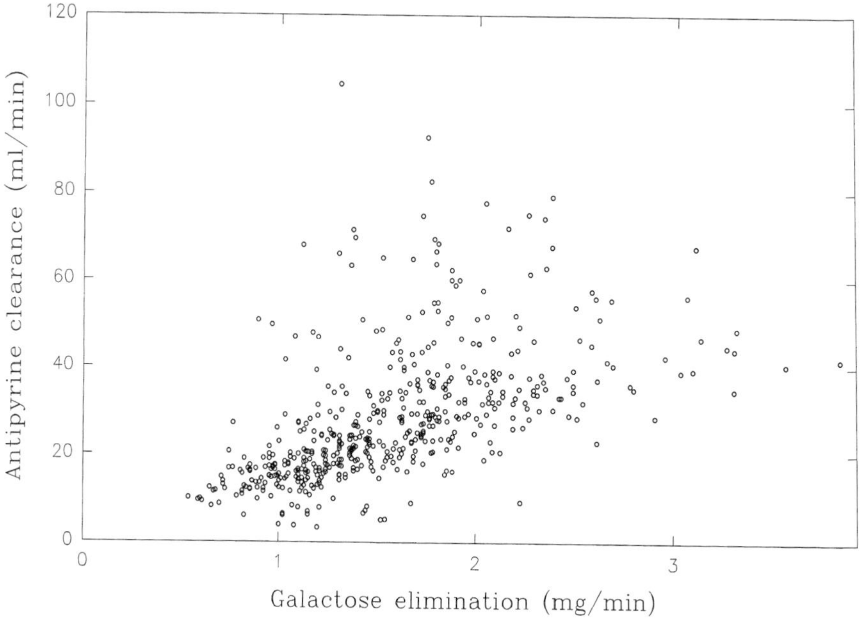

Fig. 2 Relation between antipyrine clearance and galactose elimination capacity in patients with liver disease ($n = 518$; $r = 0.54$.)

be because different functions are not similarly suppressed in liver damage. Whether one or more of these causes have had an influence on one or both of the tests compared remains unknown. The question of which is the better test cannot be answered.

Test results have also been evaluated by their correlation with commonly accepted measures of severity, such as histological or clinical scores. Histological scores have the problem of quantification and representativeness, and a correlation with clinical scores does not answer whether the test or the score is the better indicator of severity. Since the clinical score may be easier and cheaper than the test the result of the analysis will be of little practical value.

SURROGATES FOR PROGNOSIS

The clinical interest in quantitative liver tests is motivated by the expectation that the severity of liver dysfunction is closely related to the prognosis. Absolute prognostic information from a quantitative liver function test is only possible if: (1) the test quantifies the relevant function; (2) the event always occurs at the same level of that function; and (3) the function changes linearly, always with the same slope. An animal model has indicated approximation to this situation[5]. A similar situation has not been demonstrated in patients, nor is it likely to exist.

To relate a test to prognosis requires a definition of prognosis, often including a specification of the intended gain from treatment. Prognosis is quantified as the probability for a given event to occur within a given period of time. Evidence for prognostic information is statistical in nature.

In fulminant hepatitis, for example, it may be relatively simple to define prognosis, viz. the short-term survival. Several tests indicating the chance of survival are used. Even in this case, where a number of factors other than liver function, such as aetiology, age, complications etc. may have great influence, a very close relation between a quantitative test and prognosis should not be expected.

For the long-term prognosis of chronic liver disease the relation will be weaker because uncertainty increases with time and the effect of 'confounding' factors may increase. Furthermore, it will depend on the endpoint selected. Data indicating risk of variceal haemorrhage are not identical to those indicating risk of death[6], even if the endpoints are associated.

A large number of clinical and laboratory variables have been shown by univariate analysis to be related to prognosis, especially survival, in patients with chronic liver disease. Demonstration of such a relation does not prove that a test provides new prognostic information, not obtained by other, simpler means.

The simpler means may be routine clinical and laboratory observations which still are valid, and appreciation that a combination of observations may contain more than one piece of information. The combination suggested by Child and Turcotte, later modified by Pugh, here referred to as Child class or Child score, is widely and increasingly used to describe severity as well as prognosis, and is widely accepted as a 'gold standard'.

Multiple regression analysis has now made more rational approaches possible for evaluation of prognostic information from all available information. The method accepts that factors other than liver function *per se* may play a role. Furthermore, it ranks observations according to weight, ensuring proportionality to the prognostic endpoint, and it eliminates observations which contain essentially the same information as the most significant one. The Child score neglects these factors[7], and multiple regression analysis should be preferred to evaluate the prognostic significance of quantitative tests. The validation is not complete, however, until the results have been confirmed in prospective studies, which is rarely the case.

TESTS

A number of the available, commonly used tests are discussed below, in the light of recent studies.

Aminopyrine breath test

This is probably the most used quantitative liver function test. It is relatively easy and cheap to perform, and the amount of radioactivity administered is considered to be harmless. Several steps are involved between the metabolism of the compound and exhalation of radioactive carbon dioxide. The kinetics are not well understood, and it is uncertain whether the capacity of the hepatic metabolism is saturated.

Several clinical studies have confirmed a correlation with other quantitative tests and with survival by univariate analysis. Studies comparing the test with the Child classes have given variable results. Two found the test clearly inferior[8,9], one[10] found no additive value of the test, and in one[11], the test could discriminate between two prognostic groups in class B. A study using multivariate regression analysis[12] found that the test had a (slightly) more significant contribution to an index for death in liver failure than the score. Among the components of the score, only ascites and bilirubin contributed significantly. The test has been suggested to be useful for selecting liver recipients[13]. However, to our knowledge, no transplantation centre has used a quantitative test as the only or main criterion. Rejection episodes in transplanted patients transiently reduced the test result, concomitantly with changes in alanine aminotransferase levels[14].

Antipyrine clearance test

This test is easy and cheap to administer, but analysis of the compound requires a well equipped laboratory. The metabolism and elimination kinetics are known, the clearance is 'intrinsic', i.e. V_{max}/K_m, independent of the hepatic flow, and thus a measure of the capacity of the function, provided that K_m is always the same. As a self-administered, saliva one-sample test it lends itself to frequent out-patient or home follow-up studies. Side-effects of antipyrine, seen after therapeutic use of the drug, have not been seen after the test dose.

A correlation with liver mass after partial hepatectomy has been demonstrated in rats, but not all of the metabolic pathways are reduced to the same extent in experimental cirrhosis[15]. Antipyrine clearance is correlated with other quantitative tests in patients and control subjects, but as shown in Figure 2, greatly deviating values are frequent.

We have followed a group of patients with primary biliary cirrhosis for a long period of time with this test, hoping to be able to demonstrate the gradual downhill course characteristic of this disease. It was not possible to show a relation between spikes or troughs of the curves and clinical developments in individual patients. Similar variations were not seen in the galactose elimination capacity (Figure 3). On the other hand, in patients followed until death a preceding decline was noted.

Caffeine clearance test

This test can also be performed as a non-invasive, self-administered test[16], and it is correlated with the aminopyrine breath test. Experimental data in rats have confirmed agreement between *in vitro* and *in vivo* intrinsic clearance and V_{max}[17], supporting the fact that caffeine clearance is a measure of capacity. It is influenced by the state of the P450 system, especially the intake of coffee, probably accounting for the wide range seen in control subjects. The systemic clearance is higher than for antipyrine; an influence of hepatic blood flow is therefore likely.

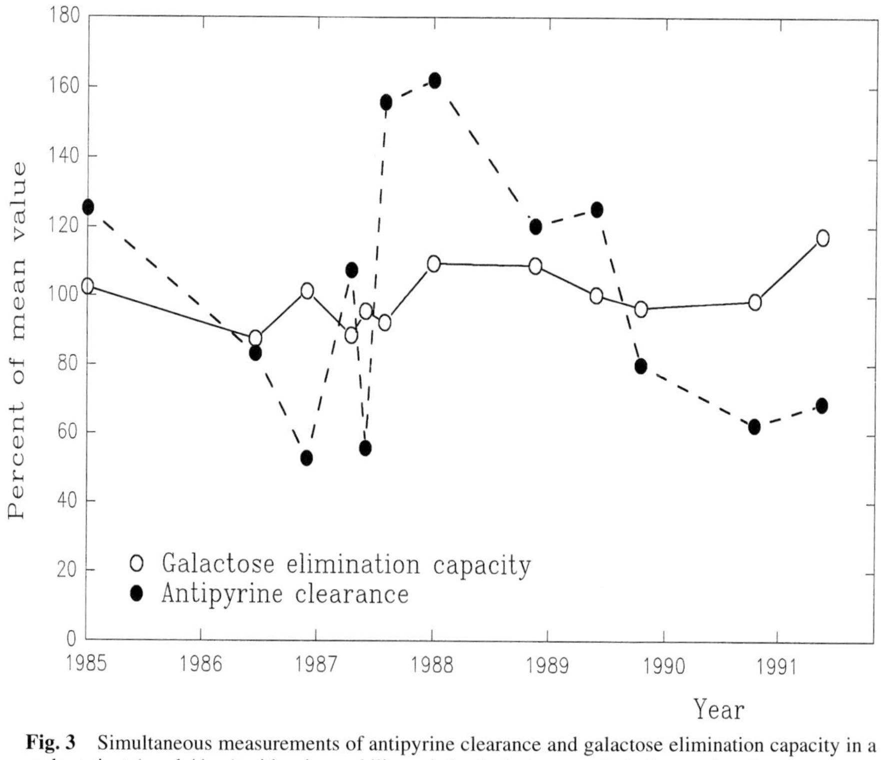

Fig. 3 Simultaneous measurements of antipyrine clearance and galactose elimination capacity in a male patient (aged 41 yr) with primary biliary cirrhosis during a period of more than 6 years

Caffeine clearance has been found to be related to survival in cirrhotic patients[18]. The test had little value in detection of rejection in a small group of transplanted patients[19].

MEGX test

This test measures the blood level of monoethylglycinexylidide (MEGX), a lidocaine metabolite shortly after intravenous injection of the compound. The short test period is an advantage for assessment of the functional integrity of donor livers. It shares with other drug tests a dependence on the status of the P450 system. It reflects lidocaine clearance and is correlated with systemic indocyanine clearance, both of which are dependent on the hepatic blood flow.

In patients with cirrhosis from Taiwan, good correlation between MEGX and systemic indocyanine green clearance and galactose elimination was found[20]; the correlation was less with Child scores. Univariate analysis showed relation with survival. A simultaneous study in European patients with liver disease found lower, although significant, correlations with Child scores[21]. The aminopyrine breath test discriminated better among patients with increasing severity than MEGX, while galactose elimination capacity discriminated better between mild liver disease and cirrhosis.

Multiple regression analysis showed that the MEGX test added significantly to a model including Child scores[22], and a low MEGX test was considered a more reliable indicator of risk for developing liver failure[23]. In a large group of patients with chronic hepatitis, half with cirrhosis, the MEGX test showed decreasing, though overlapping, values with increasing histologic severity (Knodell score), inversely related to ALT values during treatment[24]. The test was significantly reduced in cirrhotic patients, and Child class C patients had significantly lower values than A and B.

The MEGX test has been proposed for assessment of donor livers as significantly lower values have been found in grafts surviving less than 120 days[25]. In a later study early graft function was better in donor livers with high MEGX values, but graft survival was not significantly related to it[26].

Indocyanine clearance tests

This test, performed by a single intravenous injection of indocyanine green, and following blood concentrations in blood samples or by ear oximetry, measures the systemic clearance of the compound. The high clearance makes it very dependent of hepatic blood flow which has been considered an advantage[22]. By univariate analysis a relation to prognosis in cirrhotic patients has been shown[18]. The test did not predict survival or encephalopathy following porto–caval shunt surgery[27], but it contributed significantly to a regression model, including Child scores[22]. Transplant recipients with donor livers with low indocyanine green clearance showed greater postoperative impairment in prothrombin value, and primary non-function was (not significantly) more frequent[28].

The intrinsic indocyanine clearance (V_{max}/K_m), which requires hepatic venous blood measurement and is flow independent, was only weakly correlated with three of the components of the Child score, considered to indicate the score is not the best indicator of impairment of liver function[29]. The test was a significant predictor of survival in cirrhosis by univariate analysis[30] but did not contribute to a multivariate model containing only ascites and albumin.

Galactose elimination capacity

This test differs from the above by loading with a physiological compound, although in unphysiological concentrations. It is invasive, requiring intravenous injection and sampling of (capillary) blood. The only complication is from perivenous injection by mistake. It is assumed to measure the capacity for galactose phosphorylation, which again may depend on availability of ATP[31]. The kinetics in the liver are well described; some extrahepatic removal is likely, but probably constant[32], i.e. independent of liver function. A relation to liver volume has been shown experimentally in rats following partial hepatectomy[2] and following porto–caval shunt[33].

Clinical studies have given variable results. By univariate analysis the galactose test was significantly related to survival, but not included in the model by multivariate analysis after the Child score[8]. In a similarly designed study[34] the galactose test was included in the model after the Child score and in a model after inclusion of the three significant components of the score, i.e. albumin, bilirubin and encephalopathy. Consecutive tests did not predict later development in a mixed population of cirrhotic patients[35], but indicated improvement in abstaining alcoholics, as also observed by others. In primary biliary cirrhosis a decline in the test result predicted fatal outcome earlier than the Mayo model[36], which could be substituted by a model including only bilirubin and galactose elimination. In a randomized trial of interferon treatment of chronic hepatitis B[37], the galactose test deteriorated only in patients who did not become HBV DNA negative.

Urea synthesis rate

Urea synthesis rate depends on, among several other factors, the amino acid concentration in the blood. From measurement of synthesis at different amino acid concentrations, obtained by intravenous injection, a ratio (the functional hepatic nitrogen clearance) may be determined. It is reduced in patients with cirrhosis, and correlated with the galactose elimination capacity[38]. A simpler procedure has been suggested[39], but still the method is probably more demanding than most clinicians will accept for routine use. If further validation is satisfactory the test may be a candidate for the 'gold standard' status, in which case a certain amount of complexity must be accepted.

CONCLUSION

Despite numerous studies progress on quantification of liver function has been slow. The number of tests is growing; they differ with respect to secondary characteristics such as cost, time required, side-effects etc., but not one distinguishes itself as the test of choice, suggesting general recommendation or nomination as the gold standard.

The lack of a gold standard is a key problem. To find one much more must be known about liver function in health and disease. Answers are more likely to come from basic than from clinical science. Molecular biology, which has had such a great impact on many other aspects of hepatology, may give a clue. Possibly a set of gold standards is needed, dependent on the clinical situation, i.e. the pathogenesis of the disease and the endpoint studied.

Clinical science is responsible for exploration of the prognostic return from quantitative liver function estimates, those existing as well as future tests. Multivariate regression analysis appears to be the most powerful tool for this job, especially the time dependent model, which operates with shorter time intervals and can take unforeseen events in account. Such studies may be conducted as randomized therapeutic trials, which permit comparison of the contribution of several quantitative tests to therapeutic indices. It is important, however, that the studies comprise sufficiently large, homogeneous groups of patients, and well defined, clinically relevant endpoints. Probably multicentre studies will be necessary.

Unfortunately studies of this kind have a high cost/benefit ratio, where the cost is time and careful work needed, and benefit is scientific merit for the workers. This applies even more to the equally important next step, viz. validation of the results in prospective studies. A possible solution may be that health care administrators are increasingly interested in informatics and quality control, and therefore will be willing to provide the investments which make the enterprise feasible.

The problems of quantifying liver function are still unsolved, and to develop and evaluate quantitative tests remains a major challenge for hepatologists involved in both basic and clinical science.

References

1. Bachmann KA, Jauregui L. Use of single sample clearance estimates of cytochrome P450 substrates to characterize human hepatic CYP status *in vivo*. Xenobiotica. 1993;23:307–15.
2. Hansen BA, Poulsen HE. Changes in the hepatic capacity of urea-N synthesis, galactose elimination and antipyrine clearance following 70% hepatectomy in the rat. Scand J Clin Lab Invest. 1986;46:233–7.
3. Reichen J, Arts B, Schafroth U, Zimmermann A, Zeltner Th, Zysset T. Aminopyrine N-demethylation by rats with liver cirrhosis: Evidence for the intact cell hypothesis. A morphometric-functional study. Gastroenterology. 1987;93:719–26.
4. Kawasaki S, Imamura H, Bandai Y, Sanjo K, Idezuki Y. Direct evidence for the intact hepatocyte theory in patients with liver cirrhosis. Gastroenterology. 1992;102:1351–5.
5. Gross JB, Reichen J, Zeltner TB, Zimmermann A. The evolution of changes in quantitative liver function tests in a rat model of biliary cirrhosis: Correlation with morphometric measurement of hepatocyte mass. Hepatology. 1987;7:457–63.
6. Gluud C, Henriksen JH, Nielsen G, CSL. Prognostic indicators in alcoholic cirrhotic men. Hepatology. 1988;8:222–7.
7. Christensen, E, Schlichting P, Fauerholdt L *et al.* Prognostic value of Child–Turcotte criteria in medically treated cirrhosis. Hepatology. 1984;4:430–5.
8. Albers I, Hartmann H, Bircher J, Creutzfeldt W. Superiority of the Child–Pugh classification to quantitative liver function tests for assessing prognosis of liver cirrhosis. Scand J Gastroenterol. 1989;24:269–76.
9. Beuers, U, Jager F, Wahllander A, Ansari H, Kirsch CM. Prognostic value of the intravenous 14C-aminopyrine breath test compared to the Child–Pugh score and serum bile acids in 84 cirrhotic patients. Digestion. 1991;50:3–4.

10. Villeneuve J-P, Infante-Rivard C, Ampelas M, Pomier-Layrargues G, Huet P-M, Marleau D. Prognostic value of the aminopyrine breath test in cirrhotic patients. Hepatology. 1986;6:928–31.
11. Urbain D, Muls V, Thys O, Ham HR. Aminopyrine breath test improves long-term prognostic evaluation in patients with alcoholic cirrhosis in Child classes A and B. J Hepatol. 1995;22:179–83.
12. Merkel C, Bolognesi M, Bellon S *et al.* Aminopyrine breath test in the prognostic evaluation of patients with cirrhosis. Gut. 1992;33:836–42.
13. Aran P, Kane S, Baker AL. Aminopyrine breath test measurements in the evaluation of liver transplantation outcome. Hepatology. 1989;10:570.
14. Heidecke CD, Martin WG, Muller DF *et al.* Acute liver allograft rejection and liver function: quantitative evaluation using the [14C]aminopyrine breath test. Transplant Proc. 1993 Aug;25(4):2640–1.
15. Buters JTM, Zysset T, Reichen J. Metabolism of antipyrine *in vivo* in two rat models of liver cirrhosis. Its relationship to intrinsic clearance *in vitro* and microsomal membrane lipid composition. Biochem Pharmacol. 1993;46:983–91.
16. Jost G, Wahlländer A, Mandach Uv, Preisig R. Overnight salivary caffeine clearance: A liver function test suitable for routine use. Hepatology. 1987;7:338–44.
17. Hayes KA, Brennan B, Chenery R, Houston JB. *In vivo* disposition of caffeine predicted from hepatic microsomal and hepatocyte data. Drug Metab Dispos. 1995;23:349–53.
18. Lautz HU, Schmidt FW, Schmidt E, Müller MJ, Balint J. Quantitative liver function tests as predictors of survival in hepatic and primary biliary cirrhosis. Hepatology, 1988;8:1414.
19. Nagel RA, Dirix LY, Hayllar KM, Preisig R, Tredger JM, Williams R. Use of quantitative liver function tests – caffeine clearance and galactose elimination capacity – after orthotopic liver transplantation. J Hepatol. 1990 Mar;10(2):149–57.
20. Huang YS, Lee SD, Deng JF *et al.* Measuring lidocaine metabolite – monoethylglycinexylidide as a quantitative index of hepatic function in adults with chronic hepatitis and cirrhosis. J Hepatol. 1993 Aug;19(1):140–7.
21. Meyer-Wyss B, Renner E, Luo H, Scholer A. Assessment of lidocaine metabolite formation in comparison with other quantitative liver function tests. J Hepatol. 1993;19:133–9.
22. Oellerich M, Burdelski M, Lautz H-U, Binder L, Pichlmayr R. Predictors of one-year pretransplant survival in patients with cirrhosis. Hepatology. 1991;14:1029–34.
23. Arrigoni A, Gindro T, Aimo G *et al.* Monoethylglicinexylidide test: A prognostic indicator of survival in cirrhosis. Hepatology. 1994;20:383–7.
24. Shiffman ML, Luketic MA, Sanjal MJ *et al.* Hepatic lidocaine metabolism and liver histology in patients with chronic hepatitis and cirrhosis. Hepatology. 1994;19:933–40.
25. Oellerich M, Burdelski M, Ringe B *et al.* Lignocaine metabolite formation as a measure of pre-transplant liver function. Lancet. 1989;1:640–2.
26. Adam R, Azoulay D, Astarcioglu I *et al.* Limits of the MEGX test in the selection of liver grafts for transplantation. Transplant Proc. 1993;25:1653–4.
27. Pomier-Layrargues G, Huet P-M, Infante-Rivard C *et al.* Prognostic value of indocyanine green and lidocaine kinetics for survival and chronic hepatic encephalopathy in cirrhotic patients following elective end-to-side portacaval shunt. Hepatology. 1988;8:1506–10.
28. Koneru B, Leevy CB, Klein KM, Zweil P, Wilson DJ. Indocyanine green clearance in the evaluation of donor livers. Transplant Proc. 1993;25:1919–20.
29. Barbare JC, Poupon RE, Jaillon P, Prod'homme S, Darnis F, Poupon RY. Intrinsic hepatic clearance and Child–Turcotte classification for assessment of liver function in cirrhosis. J Hepatol. 1985;1:253–9.
30. Merkel C, Bolognesi M, Finucci GF *et al.* Indocyanine green intrinsic clearance as a prognostic index of survival in patients with cirrhosis. J Hepatol. 1989;9:16–22.
31. Tygstrup N, Vall¢-Hansen F, T¢nnesen K, Keiding S. Kinetics of galactose metabolism in the perfused pig liver. In: Lundquist F, Tygstrup N, editors. Regulation of hepatic metabolism. Copenhagen: Munksgaard, 1974:314–23.
32. Lindskov J, Ranek L, Tygstrup N, Winkler K. Splanchnic galactose uptake in patients with cirrhosis during continuous infusion. Clin Physiol. 1983;3:179–85.
33. Lauterburg BH, Sautter V, Preisig R, Bircher J. Hepatic functional deterioration after portacaval shunt in the rat. Effects on sulfobromophthalein transport-maximum, indocyanine green clearance and galactose elimination capacity. Gastroenterology. 1976;71:221–7.

34. Merkel C, Gatta A, Zoli M *et al.* Prognostic value of galactose elimination capacity, aminopyrine breath test, and ICG clearance in patients with cirrhosis. Comparison with the Pugh score. Dig Dis Sci. 1991 Sep;36(9):1197–203.
35. Marchesini G, Fabbri A, Bugianesi E *et al.* Analysis of the deterioration rates of liver function in cirrhosis, based on galactose elimination capacity. Liver. 1990;10:65–71.
36. Reichen J, Widmer T, Cotting J. Accurate prediction of death by serial determination of galactose elimination capacity in primary biliary cirrhosis: A comparison with the Mayo model. Hepatology. 1991;14:504–10.
37. Reichen J, Bianchi L, Frei PC, Male PJ, Lavanchy D, Schmid M, Swiss Association for the Study of the Liver. Efficacy of steroid withdrawal and low-dose interferon treatment in chronic active hepatitis B. Results of a randomized multicenter trial. J Hepatol. 1994 Feb;20(2):168–74.
38. Vilstrup H. Synthesis of urea after stimulation with amino acids: relation to liver function. Gut. 1980;21:990–5.
39. Hamberg O, Vilstrup H. A rapid method for determination of hepatic amino nitrogen to urea nitrogen conversion ('the functional hepatic nitrogen clearance'). Scand J Clin Lab Invest. 1994;54:377–83.

5
The threshold hypothesis of sodium retention in the presence of liver disease provides a surrogate marker for the onset of ascites

R. A. BRANCH, R. SABRA and J. F. BERNARDO

INTRODUCTION

A surrogate marker is by definition a substitute measure for a process. For it to have value in a clinical context, this measure should be easy to obtain, be without risk to the patient and should be a reliable predictor of a clinical outcome. Preferably it should also be quantitative and not influenced by factors other than the clinical outcome it is attempting to predict.

In almost all areas of medicine, it has been possible either directly to measure the change in organ function or find a suitable surrogate marker of overall function. However, the liver has proved to be one of the most refractory areas to develop and validate reliable measures of aspects of hepatic physiology that relate to clinical complications. Despite its complexity, the liver has a limited repertoire of pathophysiological responses to a variety of disease states. These include altered hepatic acinar architecture with loss of acinar structure, a breakdown of the acinar organization and alteration in the proportions of different cell populations. As the acinar framework is disrupted, patterns and pressures of hepatic haemodynamics are altered, the relative perfusion provided by portal venous blood and the hepatic artery change, and the microcirculation is altered by the development of capillarization. Despite the variety and complexity of these functional and anatomical changes, the clinical expression of extensive liver disease is remarkably similar irrespective of the aetiology. In general, the initial clinical evidence of deteriorating liver disease is the development of ascites. Gastrointestinal haemorrhage from oesophago-gastric varices may precede this complication, and hepatic encephalopathy and bleeding diatheses may be associated with it and with even worse hepatic function. However, the most common clinical complication leading to the diagnosis of end stage liver disease is the onset of ascites. If the onset of ascites is related to extent of disease, then a valid question to raise is whether a surrogate measure of liver function could be developed that might predict whether or not the onset of this event is imminent.

In recent years, there has been considerable interest in evaluating the interrelationships of physiologically independent parameters of hepatic function. Our interest was stimulated by considering the implications of the physiological determinants of drug disposition[1]. It is now well established that drugs exclusively cleared by the liver with a low intrinsic clearance have liver blood flow-independent kinetics. Conversely, drugs that are also exclusively cleared by the liver but have a high intrinsic clearance are liver blood flow dependent[2]. Thus, simultaneous measurement of two such model probes should be able to discriminate between changes in function and flow. Interestingly, a number of studies from various laboratories including our own have shown close correlations between clearances of low and high clearance drugs. They include antipyrine as an example of a low clearance drug, and propranolol[3], galactose[4] and lignocaine[5], as examples of high clearance drugs. We have, therefore, developed an operational model, the intact hepatocyte theory, which assumes that even in cirrhosis, hepatic extraction is normal[6]. Thus it is assumed that the reduction in intrinsic clearance occurs because certain cells in the liver lack the relevant enzyme, whereas the rest retain a relatively normal enzyme concentration. The reduced clearance of poorly extracted drugs is attributable to the fall in intrinsic clearance, while the reduction in extraction of highly extracted drugs is considered due to the presence of functional shunts which flow through parts of the liver containing cells with little or no enzyme, thus allowing drug to escape metabolism[7].

The operational nature of this model should be stressed, however, because it is a pathological oversimplification. For example, we recognize that functional shunts will be created when vessels pass through fibrous tissue as well as perfusing hepatocytes without drug metabolizing activity. Furthermore, reduction in organ blood flow need not necessarily be shared equally among all the lobules. Given that viable hepatocytes must receive some perfusion, the central question revolves around the enzyme content of these cells. Unfortunately, because of the suggestion that the degree of functional shunting may change with altered flow, we cannot actually distinguish whether the perfused hepatocytes contain a normal or reduced amount of enzyme. Given that hepatic function and functional flow maintain a relationship, the question is, does either relate to the onset of ascites?

The role of the liver in the development of salt retention in cirrhosis is incompletely understood. Recently, the concepts explaining the onset of sodium retention and the possible involvement of the liver in its pathogenesis have changed. Despite these changes, the pivotal role of hepatic function in the regulation of renal function remains a central theme. The traditional concept was that salt retention occurs as a result of a diminished intravascular volume caused by changes in Starling forces and subsequent transudation of fluid into the abdominal cavity (classical underfilling theory)[8]. The role of the liver was limited to a mechanical block initiating the process of ascites formation. This concept was first questioned by Lieberman, Ito and Reynolds[9] and Lieberman, Denison and Reynolds[10]. Based on their findings of an increased total blood volume in cirrhotic patients, they proposed the overflow theory of ascites formation and salt retention. According to this theory, reduced hepatic function is associated with changes that result in primary renal salt and water retention[11–14]. This leads to an increased intravascular volume that, in combination with abnormal Starling forces, causes the formation of ascites as an overflow phenomenon. Thus, the crucial contribution of the liver to the pathogenesis of salt retention is functional, rather than mechanical. More recently, the findings that peripheral vasodilatation and an increase in cardiac output occur before ascites formation in cirrhosis have led to the proposal of the peripheral arterial vasodilatation hypothesis[15]. This hypothesis suggests that decreased hepatic function is associated with increased vascular capacitance that leads to decreased effective arterial blood volume. Secondary hormonal and neural changes cause the initiation of renal sodium and water retention, followed by ascites formation when compensatory mechanisms become insufficient. Again, it appears conceivable that the liver could initiate this process by decreased production or metabolism of a vasoactive factor.

Irrespective of the mechanism involved, it appears that a reduction in liver function is a major determinant of the onset of sodium retention. An inference of this observation is that measures of liver function could be used as surrogate predictors of the risk of developing ascites. Theoretically, it is possible that such a relationship or association could either be linear, similar to that between liver function and functional hepatic blood flow, or alternatively that renal homeostasis is maintained until liver function falls below a critical threshold, at which point sodium retention occurs, in which case a non-linear relationship would be anticipated (Figure 1).

In order to evaluate these alternative hypotheses in a variety of animal models, we have used the ^{14}C aminopyrine breath test (ABT) as a non-invasive, easily measured surrogate marker of hepatic function in the rat. The ABT provides a quantitative measurement of hepatic function that can be repeatedly

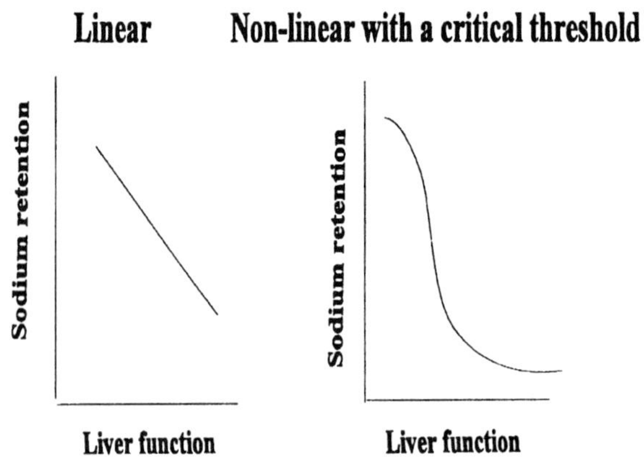

Fig. 1 Schematic representation of alternative possible relationships between liver function and renal sodium retention

measured in longitudinal studies in the rat. Hepner and Vesell[16] and Lauterburg and Bircher[17] first introduced the test as a non-invasive measure of hepatic mixed function oxidase activity *in vivo* in humans and rats. The rate of change of $^{14}CO_2$ recovered from exhaled breath in timed collections has been shown to correlate with the plasma disappearance of unchanged parent drug and the plasma elimination of the main metabolite of aminopyrine, 4-amino-antipyrine[18,19] and has also been shown to be of prognostic value[20,21]. The test has been used in rat models after induction of acute liver damage, hepatectomy and induction of cirrhosis by bile duct ligation and carbon tetrachloride (CCl_4) inhalation[6,22,23]. Reichen *et al.*[24] demonstrated that, in the rat model of CCl_4-induced cirrhosis, a reduction in aminopyrine N-demethylation rate *in vivo* is associated with a reduction in both cytochrome P450 and microsomal amino-pyrine N-demethylase activity. The ABT exhibited a significant correlation with hepatocellular volume, suggesting that the ABT provides a measure of functioning hepatocyte mass in this model of cirrhosis.

We chose to undertake our first studies in a controlled rat model, as longitudinal studies to monitor changes in liver function in relation to renal function over a wide range of disease stages are difficult to perform in cirrhotic patient populations. Cirrhosis is usually a slowly progressive disease that develops over several years[25,26]. The rate of progression is unpredictable and the course of the disease may be interrupted by phases of recovery.

In our first study, we compared ABT and sodium homeostasis over time in the phenobarbital and CCl_4 model of cirrhosis in the rat[27]. This model has been widely used to investigate hepatic and renal function abnormalities in cirrhosis[6,24,28,29]. CCl_4-treated rats show many of the features observed in cirrhotic patients, including arterial hypotension, hypervolaemia, reduced systemic vascular resistance, portal hypertension, and reduced water and salt excretion[30–33].

The model used in many previous studies is based on the inhalation of CCl_4 as originally described by McLean, McClean and Sutton[34]. The model we choose has been adapted for oral administration by Proctor and Chatamra[35]. Their original description suggests that it offers many advantages over the more traditional model. The authors reported that no deaths occurred in the development of cirrhosis and that all animals ultimately exhibited cirrhosis with ascites within 10 weeks. Once ascites had developed, withdrawal of CCl_4 did not lead to recovery. Our experience with this model was not as favourable[27]. Even with the lowest initial dose of CCl_4, we observed death in a minority of rats and 40% of rats had sudden unexplained death within the first 8 weeks. In the remaining rats, cirrhosis developed in all animals, but the time to development of decompensation was highly variable. However, this model did have the advantage that all rats surviving the first 8 weeks ultimately developed cirrhosis and the model's long interdose interval of 7 days permitted evaluation of disease parameters in a stable stage without interrupting the dosing. In this model, sodium balance was maintained until the ABT had reached an almost equivalent value in each rat (low variance at the time of sodium retention) when there was a sudden change to avid sodium retention (Figure 2). In a further series of sodium retaining rats, the carbon tetrachloride was stopped, and when the ABT returned to the same threshold there was a spontaneous diuresis. These results strongly

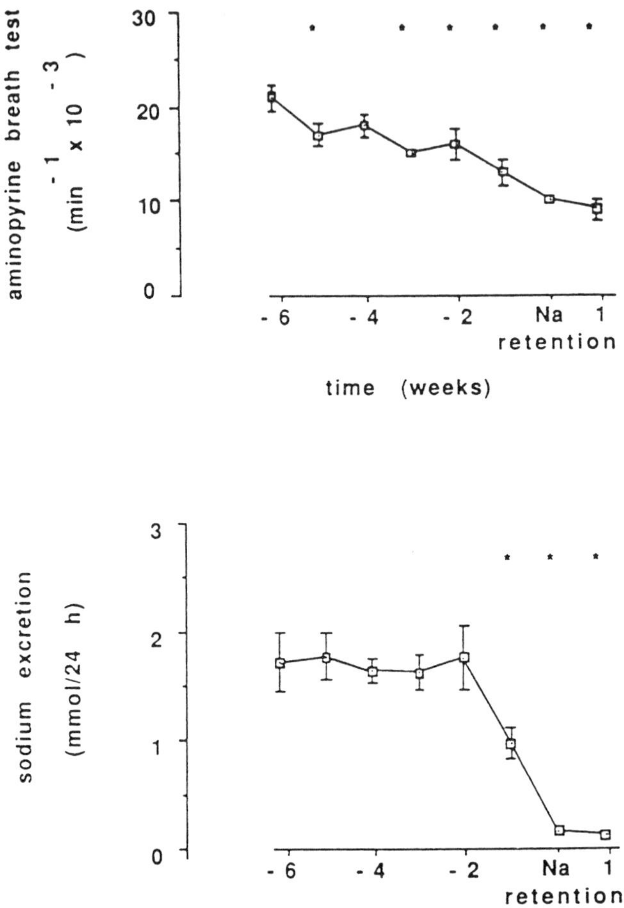

Fig. 2 Liver function and sodium excretion in chronic carbon tetrachloride model of cirrhosis in the rat. (n = 15, p <0.05 compared to week –6; time adjusted to onset of sodium retention) (from reference 27 with permission)

support the hypothesis in which liver function has to fall below a critical threshold of hepatic function to be associated with sodium retention.

If decreased catabolic or anabolic hepatic function is involved in the development of salt retention in cirrhosis, it could be anticipated that sodium retention in cirrhosis will occur at a similar degree of liver function, irrespective of the model of experimental cirrhosis. Bile duct excision is an alternative experimental model that results in cirrhosis in the rat[36,37]. It is characterized by a substantial impairment in hepatic function as assessed by the ABT[38,39], and, in contrast to the phenobarbital-carbon tetrachloride model (PB/CCl_4) of cirrhosis, does not require hepatic-enzyme induction to cause cirrhosis. We therefore designed a study to investigate the relationship between hepatic function, as assessed by the ABT, and the onset of sodium retention in this experimental model of cirrhosis, and to study whether alteration of liver function by hepatic-enzyme induction, using phenobarbital, alters this relationship[40].

In the bile duct ligated model, reductions in hepatic function, as judged by reductions in the ABT, occurred more rapidly than in the PB/CCl_4 model (Figure 3)[40]. Phenobarbital increased the ABT at all time points, but did not change its rate of change. Interestingly, sodium retention occurred at the same critical threshold in each of these three situations. One explanation for the same association between renal function and ABT in cirrhosis with or without phenobarbital is that the hepatic determinant of renal function is related to the total number of intact hepatocytes. ABT and the hepatic determinant of renal function would be similarly influenced by a decreased number of total hepatocytes in cirrhosis or a non-selective increase in functioning hepatocyte cell mass caused by phenobarbital induction.

Having shown that a similar critical threshold of hepatic function determines whether sodium homeostasis is altered in chronic models of liver disease in the rat, we next addressed whether a similar phenomenon also occurs in acute rat models. In experiments comparing sham operated rats to 1/3 partial hepatectomy and 2/3 partial hepatectomy rats in the 24 hours after surgery, we showed that when the ABT was reduced below a critical threshold, sodium retention occurred, while if the ABT was above the threshold there was no change in sodium homeostasis (Figure 4)[41]. These observations indicate that the critical threshold concept pertains irrespective of the time to achieve a given degree of hepatic dysfunction.

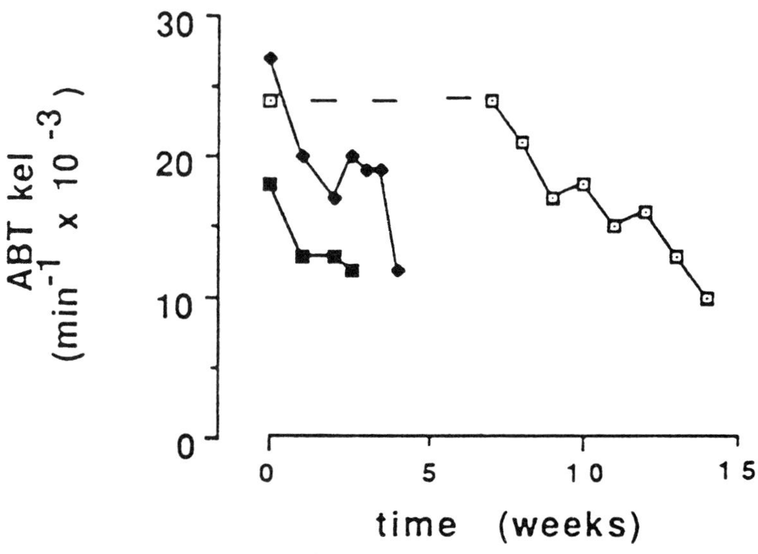

Fig. 3 Liver function to time of onset of sodium retention in chronic models of cirrhosis in the rat. ☐ Chronic CCl_4; ◆ Bile duct ligation + phenobarbital; ■ Bile duct ligation (from reference 40 with permission)

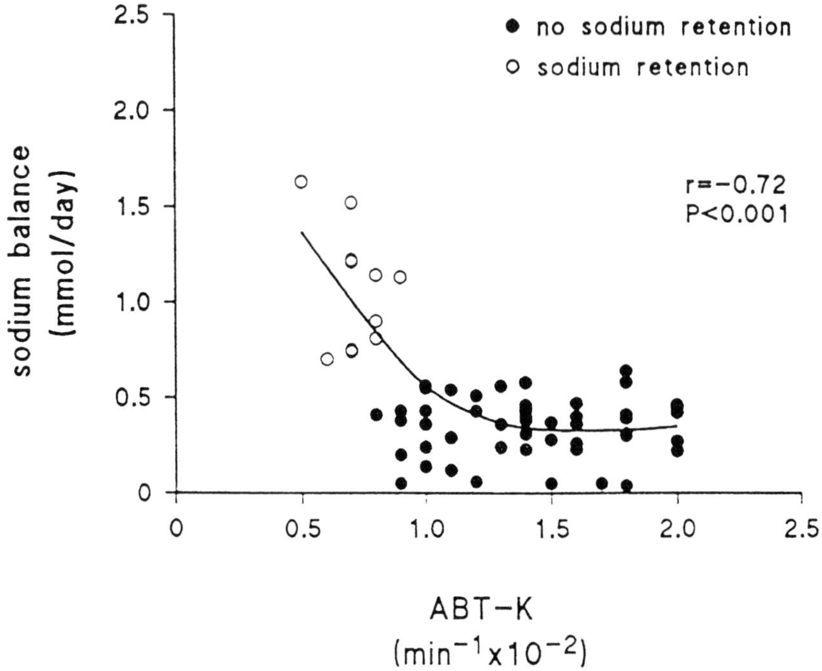

Fig. 4 Liver function and sodium balance following partial hepatectomy in the rat (from reference 41 with permission)

One potential disadvantage of each of the preceding models is that changes in hepatic function are all associated with altered portal haemodynamics, with the development of portal hypertension and a hyperdynamic circulation. In order to dissociate these changes, we used the partial portal vein ligation model where we showed that this procedure induces high sustained portal hypertension, a sustained hyperdynamic circulation, but only a transient decrease in the ABT[42]. In this model, we maintained rats on a constant sodium intake by gavage, and clearly showed that sodium retention only occurred when ABT fell below the same critical threshold that had been observed previously (Figure 5), and sodium balance was restored after the ABT returned above this threshold.

Thus, there is collectively convincing evidence that under a variety of controlled situations, the rat has a critical threshold of ABT, and irrespective of the mechanism of hepatic dysfunction, when hepatic function as measured by this surrogate marker falls below the threshold, sodium retention ensues. The reason for the association between hepatic and renal dysfunction remains unknown. We and others have taken advantage of the critical threshold concept to design experiments evaluating the contribution of a number of potential mediators of sodium retention by evaluating the level of the proposed factor or the effects of selective antagonists in rats with hepatic dysfunction with ABTs, either just above or below the critical threshold. These studies and studies in man suggest that observed changes in the sympathetic nervous system[43],

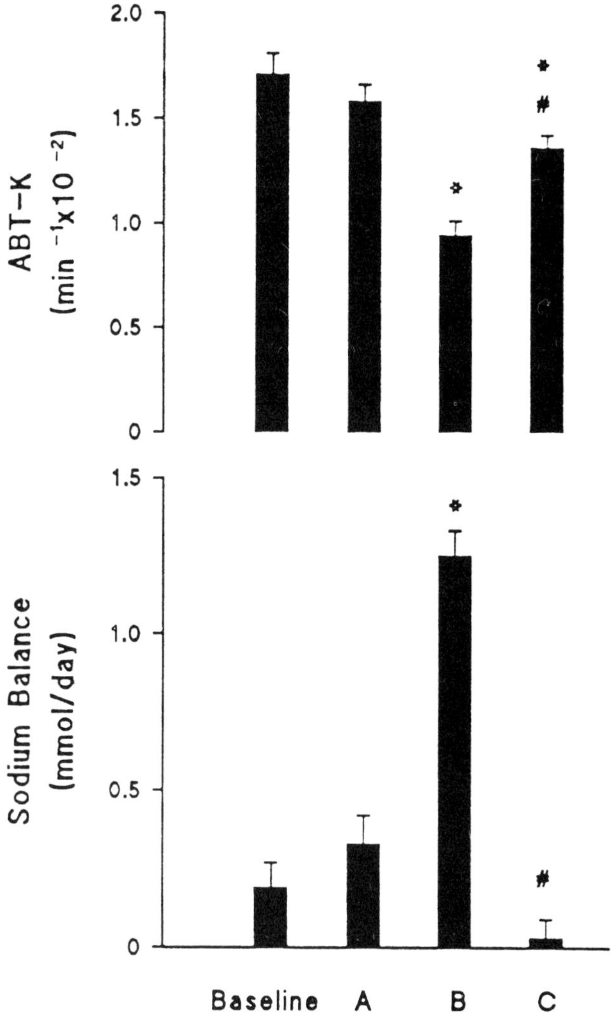

Fig. 5 Liver function and sodium balance in partial portal vein ligation model in the rat. A = day before sodium retention; B = last day of sodium retention; C = first day of natriuresis (from reference 42 with permission)

catecholamines[44,45], the renin–angiotensin–kallikrein system[46], nitric oxide production[47] and adenosine production[48] are compensatory responses, but not the prime causal agents.

Irrespective of the mechanism, there is a critical threshold of hepatic function as assessed by the ABT, below which sodium retention occurs in the rat. This concept is only relevant if a similar phenomenon can also be observed in man. This concept was first tested by Wong *et al.*[49] in man. In this study, patients with cirrhosis, but without ascites, were put on a balanced sodium intake and then challenged with a parenteral salt load. The antipyrine clearance was used as a surrogate measure of hepatic function and related to urinary sodium excretion at timed intervals following the sodium load. These authors demonstrated a positive correlation between liver function and the ability of compensated cirrhotic patients to excrete a given sodium load in their urine over 5 hours. As with aminopyrine, antipyrine elimination also depends on the activity of the hepatic mixed function oxidase enzymes. This observation implies that, with decreasing hepatic function, patients had a greater propensity to retain sodium after the salt challenge.

In a subsequent study at Erlangen, 62 unselected, stable patients hospitalized with cirrhosis were studied[50]. All subjects were free of diuretics, enzyme inducers or renal disease and were placed on a constant sodium intake (120 mmol/day) for 5 days before study. In this study, the ABT was related to 24-hour urinary sodium excretion in an unstressed situation. A curvilinear relationship similar in shape to that observed in the rat models previously described was observed. There was a critical threshold of ABT of 0.4% dose × kg/mmol CO_2 (Figure 6)[50]. The Erlangen study supports the concept of a critical threshold whereby a surrogate measure of liver function can be used to predict the risk of a patient developing ascites.

In summary, the concept that there is a critical threshold of hepatic function, as measured by its ability to undertake metabolism of aminopyrine or antipyrine, above which sodium homeostasis is normal and below which sodium retention occurs, has been demonstrated in acute and chronic models of liver disease in the rat. The same phenomenon also occurs in cirrhosis in man where both basal sodium excretion and response to a sodium challenge have been shown to relate to liver function. These observations imply that either ABT or antipyrine clear-

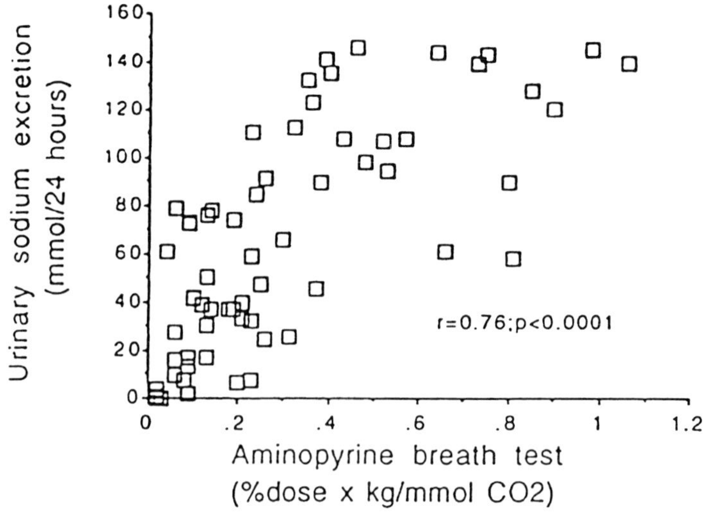

Fig. 6 Liver function and urinary sodium excretion in patients with cirrhosis (from reference 50 with permission)

ance can be used a surrogate markers to anticipate the risk of sodium retention and subsequent ascites formation. If the mechanism that coordinates functional changes in the kidney in response to decreased hepatic function could be identified, it might be possible to develop new strategies to complement sodium restriction and use of diuretics, the current mainstay of therapy.

References

1. Rowland M, Benet LZ, Graham GG. Clearance concepts in pharmacokinetics. J Pharmacokin Biopharm. 1973;1:123–36.
2. Wilkinson GR, Shand DG. Commentary: A physiological approach to hepatic drug clearance. Clin Pharmacol Ther. 1975;18:377–90.
3. Branch RA, Shand DG. Propranolol disposition in chronic liver disease: A physiological approach. Clin Pharmacokin. 1976;1:264–79.
4. Andreasson PB, Ranek L, Statland BE, Tygstrup N. Clearance of antipyrine dependence on quantitative liver function. Eur J Clin Invest. 1974;4:129–34.
5. Forrest JAH, Finlayson NDC, Adjepon-Yomoah KK, Prescott LF. Antipyrine, lignocaine and paracetamol metabolism in chronic liver disease. Gut. 1974;67:790–4.
6. Wood AJJ, Villeneuve JP, Branch RA, Roges LW, Shand DG. Intact hepatocyte theory of impaired drug metabolism in experimental cirrhosis in the rat. Gastroenterology. 1979;76:1358–62.
7. Shand DG, Branch RA, Wood AJJ, Villeneuve JP. Drug metabolism in experimental cirrhosis: The intact hepatocyte theory. In: Preisig R, Birscher J, editors. The liver quantitative aspects of structure and function. 3rd International Gstood Symposium. 1978:346–50.
8. Papper S. The role of the kidney in Laennec's cirrhosis of the liver. Medicine. 1958;37:229–316.
9. Lieberman FL, Ito S, Reynolds TB. Effective plasma volume in cirrhosis with ascites: Evidence that a decreased volume does not account for renal sodium retention, a spontaneous reduction in glomerular filtration rate (GFR), and a fall in GFR during drug-induced diuresis. J Clin Invest. 1969;48:975–81.
10. Lieberman FL, Denison EK, Reynolds TB. The relationship of plasma volume, portal hypertension, ascites and renal sodium retention in cirrhosis: The 'overflow' theory of ascites formation. Ann NY Acad Sci. 1970;170:202–6.
11. Levy M. Sodium retention and ascites formation in dogs with experimental portal cirrhosis. Am J Physiol. 1977;233:F572–85.
12. Levy M, Wexler MJ. Renal sodium retention and ascites formation in dogs with experimental cirrhosis but without portal hypertension or increased splanchnic vascular capacity. J Lab Clin Med. 1978;91:520–36.
13. Lopez-Novoa JM, Rengel MA, Hernando L. Dynamics of ascites formation in rats with experimental cirrhosis. Am J Physiol. 1980;238:F353–7.
14. Jimenez W, Martinez-Pardo A, Arroyo V *et al.* Temporal relationship between hyperaldosteronism, sodium retention, and ascites formation in rats with experimental cirrhosis. Hepatology. 1985;5:245–50.
15. Schrier RW, Arroyo V, Bernardi M, Epstein M, Henrikson JH, Rodés J. Peripheral arterial vasodilation hypothesis: A proposal for the initiation of renal sodium and water retention in cirrhosis. Hepatology. 1988;8:1151–7.
16. Hepner GW, Vesell ES. Quantitative assessment of hepatic function by breath analysis after oral administration of (14C) aminopyrine. N Engl J Med. 1974;291:1384–7.
17. Lauterburg BH, Bircher J. Expiratory measurement of maximal aminopyrine demethylation *in vivo*: Effect of phenobarbital, partial hepatectomy, porto-caval shunt, and bile duct ligation in the rat. J Pharmacol Exp Ther. 1976;196:501–9.
18. Hepner GW, Vesell ES. Aminopyrine disposition: Studies on breath, saliva and urine of normal subjects and patients with liver disease. Clin Pharmacol Ther. 1976;20:654–60.
19. Bircher J, Küpfer A, Gikalov I, Preisig R. Aminopyrine demethylation measured by breath analysis in cirrhosis. Clin Pharmacol Ther. 1976;20:484–92.

20. Schneider JF, Baker AL, Haines NM, Hatfield G, Boyer JL. Aminopyrine N-demethylation: A prognostic test of liver function in patients with alcoholic liver disease. Gastroenterology. 1980;79:1145–50.
21. Gill RA, Goodman MW, Golfus GR, Onstad GR, Bubrick MP. Aminopyrine breath tests predicts surgical risk for patients with liver disease. Ann Surg. 1983;198:701–4.
22. Gross JB, Reichen R, Zeltner TB, Zimmermann A. The evolution of changes in quantitative liver function tests in rat model of biliary cirrhosis: Correlation with morphometric measurement of hepatocyte mass. Hepatology. 1987;7:457–63.
23. Sendama I, De Hemptinne B, Lambotte L. Recovery of liver function in partially hepatectomized rats evaluated by aminopyrine demethylation capacity. Hepatology. 1985;5:629–33.
24. Reichen J, Arts B, Schafroth U, Zimmermann A, Zeltner B, Zysett T. Aminopyrine N-demethylation by rats with liver cirrhosis. Gastroenterology. 1987;93:719–26.
25. Klinger EL Jr, Vaamonde CA, Vammonde LS *et al.* Renal function changes in cirrhosis of the liver. Arch Intern Med. 1970;125:1010–5.
26. Gabudzda GJ. Cirrhosis, ascites and edema: clinical course related to management. Gastroenterology. 1970;58:546–53.
27. Wensing G, Sabra R, Branch RA. The onset of sodium retention in experimental cirrhosis in rats is related to a critical threshold of liver function. Hepatology. 1990;11:779–86.
28. Gross JB, Reichen R, Zeltner TB, Zimmermann A. The evolution of changes in quantitative liver function tests in rat model of biliary cirrhosis: Correlation with morphometric measurement of hepatocyte mass. Hepatology. 1987;7:457–63.
29. Reichen J, Egger B, Ohara N, Zeltner TB, Zysset T, Simmermann A. Determinations of hepatic function in liver cirrhosis. J Clin Invest. 1988;82:2069–76.
30. Lopez-Novoa JM, Rengel MA, Rodicio JL, Hernando L. Micropuncture study of salt and water retention in chronic experimental cirrhosis. Am J Physiol. 1977;232:F315–8.
31. Lopez-Novoa JM, Rengel MA, Hernando L. Dynamics of ascites formation in rats with experimental cirrhosis. Am J Physiol. 1980;138:F353–7.
32. Linas SL, Anderson RJ, Guggenheim SJ, Robertson GL, Berl T. Role of vasopressin in impaired water excretion in conscious rats with experimental cirrhosis. Kidney Int. 1981;20:173–80.
33. Jimenez W, Martinez-Pardo A, Arroyo V *et al.* Temporal relationship between hyper-aldosteronism, sodium retention and ascites formation in rats with experimental cirrhosis. Hepatology. 1985;5:245–50.
34. McLean EK, McLean AEM, Sutton PM. Instant cirrhosis: An improved method for producing cirrhosis of the liver in rats by simultaneous administration of carbon tetrachloride and phenobarbitone. Br J Exp Pathol. 1969;50:502–6.
35. Proctor E, Chatamra K. High yield micronodular cirrhosis in the rat. Gastroenterology. 1982;83:1183–90.
36. Lee SS, Girod C, Braillon A, Hadengue A, Lebrec D. Hemodynamic characterization of chronic bile duct-ligated rats: Effects of phenobarbital sodium. Am J Physiol. 1986;251(2 Pt 1):G176–80.
37. Yarger WE, Schrader NW, Boyd MA. Intrarenal mechanisms of salt retention after bile duct ligation in rats. J Clin Invest. 1976;57:408–418.
38. Gross JB, Reichen R, Zeltner TB, Zimmermann A. The evolution of changes in quantitative liver function tests in rat model of biliary cirrhosis: Correlation with morphometric measurement of hepatocyte mass. Hepatology. 1987;7:457–63.
39. Lauterburg BH, Bircher J. Expiratory measurement of maximal aminopyrine demethylation *in vivo*: Affect of phenobarbital, partial hepatectomy, portocaval shunt, and bile duct ligation in the rat. J Pharmacol Exp Ther. 1976;196:501–9.
40. Wensing G, Branch RA. Phenobarbital influences the onset of sodium retention in liver disease induced by bile duct ligation in the rat. Hepatology. 1990;11:773–8.
41. Ohno T, Sabra R, Branch RA. Sodium retention and hepatic function after two thirds partial hepatectomy in the rat. Hepatology. 1991;14:511–7.
42. Ohno T, Branch RA, Sabra R. Sodium retention and hepatic function following partial portal vein ligation in the rat. J Hepatology. 1995;18:235–43.
43. Murakami S, Ohno T, Bernardo JF *et al.* Reduced liver function is the trigger for renal sodium retention following portal vein ligation in the rat. J Gastroenterol Hepatol. 1996; (in press).

44. Ring-Larsen H, Hesse B, Henriksen J, Christensen N. Sympathetic nervous activity and renal and systemic hemodynamics in cirrhosis: Plasma norepinephrine concentration, hepatic extraction and renal release. Hepatology. 1982;252:304–10.
45. Wensing G, Sabra R, Branch RA. Relationship between oxidative hepatic metabolism, urinary sodium excretion and sympathetic nerve activity in experimental cirrhosis in the rat. Z Gastroenterol. 1995;33:1–4.
46. Nicholls K, Shapiro M, Van Putten V *et al.* Elevated plasma norepinephrine concentrations in decompensated cirrhosis. Association with increased secretion rates, normal clearance rates and suppressibility of central volume expansion. Circ Res. 1985;56:457–61.
47. Murakami S, Bernardo JF, Jacob TD, Branch RA, Sabra R. Nitric oxide does not contribute to sodium retention and peripheral vasodilation induced by partial portal vein ligation in rats. Renal Physiol Biochem. 1995;18:198–208.
48. Murakami S, Bernardo JF, Branch RA, Sabra R. Adenosine does not mediate renal sodium retention and peripheral vasodilation elicited by partial portal vein ligation in rats. Hepatology. 1996;23:346–52.
49. Wong F, Massie D, Hsu P, Dudley F. Renal response to a saline load in well-compensated alcoholic cirrhosis. Hepatology. 1994;20:873–81.
50. Wensing G, Loterer E, Ahlsdorf H, Kugler CFA, Hahn EG, Fleig WE. Relationship of the aminopyrine breath test and the Child Pugh score to urinary sodium retention in patients with liver cirrhosis. Z Gastroenterol. 1995;33:150–4.

6
Scores in different diseases: a critical review and evaluation of different surrogate markers for assessing treatments in chronic liver disease

E. CHRISTENSEN and M. R. SCHUNCK

In chronic liver disease the optimal therapy should be able to stop the disease process, allowing the patient to restore functions to regain a normal life expectancy without symptoms. Treatments should preferably be assessed by studying their effects on the occurrence of hard endpoints such as death (survival analysis) in randomized clinical trials. Semi-hard endpoints such as complications (gastrointestinal bleeding, coma, decompensation) may be useful in special situations. However, many cases of chronic liver disease develop slowly, meaning that courses of diseases may be of very long duration (e.g. 5, 10 or 20 years) before any hard or semi-hard endpoint occurs. Therefore, if assessment of treatments should rely only on the study of their effects on the occurrence of hard or semi-hard endpoints, controlled clinical trials may need to be of very long duration. This would imply a rather slow development in the therapeutic field in identifying new, more effective therapies.

Hence there is a need for markers which at the earlier stages can describe the degree of progression of the disease. Chronic liver diseases have many different manifestations and therefore very many different markers may be used in theory. However, the different manifestations or markers may vary considerably in their relation to the outcome of the disease. Some disease markers may be directly related to the main disease process and to the outcome, while others may be less relevant secondary or side phenomena not related to the outcome. Only the former category of markers will be useful because such markers are related directly to the symptoms and the prognosis. However, it should be remembered that such markers are substitute or surrogate indicators of the real course of disease best being described by the occurrence of hard endpoints. Hence the term surrogate markers.

To identify variables being useful as surrogate markers one needs to analyse statistically the relation between the variables and the chosen endpoint which they should predict. A single variable is rarely sufficient. In most cases a combination of variables is needed. Therefore, multivariate statistical analyses are necessary to identify the most informative variables and describe how they should be combined to a prognostic index or score to give the best possible prediction of the endpoint in new patients.

Since such analyses are – to some degree – exploratory or heuristic, the results need some kind of validation before they can be considered to be proved. Optimally the prognostic index should be validated using the data of independent patients to see if the prognostic index in these patients predicts prognosis correctly in these patients. If completely independent patients are not available, a validation in a more limited sense can be obtained by dividing the original patient data into a 'model sample' used for the statistical development of the prognostic index and a 'test sample' used for testing and validation of the prognostic index.

In this chapter we will review and critically evaluate different surrogate markers for assessing treatments in various chronic liver diseases.

GENERAL SCORES IN CIRRHOSIS

In 1964 Child and Turcotte published their empirical criteria for assessment of hepatocellular functional reserve[1], as shown in Table 1. They comprise 5 variables (serum bilirubin, serum albumin, ascites, neurological disorder and nutrition). For a given patient each of the 5 variables is graded A, B or C scored as 1, 2 or 3, respectively, and then the points are added to give a combined score between 5 and 15. The A, B and C categories for the combined score have not been generally agreed upon[2].

Pugh *et al.*[3] have proposed a modification of the Child–Turcotte criteria in which nutrition is replaced by the prothrombin time graded as follows: 1–4 s prolonged: A; 4–6 s, prolonged: B; >6 s, prolonged: C. They define the following A, B and C grading for the combined score: 5–6: A; 7–9: B; 10–15: C[3].

Table 1 The Child–Turcotte criteria

		Group designation		
		A *1*	*B* *2*	*C* *3*
Serum bilirubin	(mg%)	<2	2–3	>3
	(μmol/L)	<34	34–51	>51
Serum albumin	(g%)	>3.5	3.0–3.5	<3.0
	(μmol/L)	>532	456–532	<456
Ascites		None	Easily controlled	Poorly controlled
Neurological disorder		None	Minimal	Advanced 'coma'
Nutrition		Good	Fair	Poor

From Child and Turcotte[1]

Although others have confirmed that the Child–Turcotte criteria hold some prognostic information[4,5], they are not optimal for several reasons: the cut-off points for categories A, B and C are completely arbitrary and not optimal; the variables are considered additive and given similar weights in the combined score; and other important prognostic variables (e.g. age) are not included. Prognostic indices based on statistical analyses have been shown to predict prognosis better[4,6]. Nevertheless, the Child–Turcotte criteria and the Pugh modification are still widely used, probably because they are quite simple to apply and because other better prognostic models have achieved less publicity and, incorrectly, are considered difficult to use.

In 1983 the Copenhagen Study Group for Liver Diseases reported the results of a Cox regression analysis of the data of 488 patients with cirrhosis[7]. The following eight variables had a significant prognostic effect: sex, age, prothrombin, acetylcholinesterase, eosinophil leukocytes in liver parenchyma, liver cell necrosis, inflammation in liver connective tissue, and efferent veins in parenchymal nodules. The variables could be combined into a prognostic index which was validated using a split sample technique.

D'Amico *et al.*.[8] found in a series of 1155 consecutive patients the following prognostic variables in compensated patients: male sex, HBsAg positivity, high age, prothrombin time prolongation, and oesophageal varices. In decompensated disease the following variables were significantly associated with a poor prognosis: hepatocellular carcinoma, encephalopathy, haemorrhage, high SGOT, oesophageal varices, high gamma-globulins, prothrombin time prolongation, continued abuse of alcohol, HBsAg positivity, high gamma-glutamyl transpeptidase, and low cholinesterase. A simple prognostic index based upon the relative risk coefficient of the significant variables was suggested but the model was not validated in independent patients.

Gines *et al.*[9] found in 293 consecutive patients with compensated cirrhosis the following variables to be associated with a poor prognosis: high serum bilirubin, high serum gamma-globulin concentration, hepatic stigmata, prolonged prothrombin time, sex, high age and high alkaline phosphatase. A prognostic index was constructed that allows calculation of the estimated survival probability. The predicting value of this index was validated by a split sample testing technique.

Based on statistical analysis of admission and follow-up data of a large number of patients with cirrhosis of mixed aetiology[10] the prognostic index presented in Table 2 was obtained. It comprises the following variables being associated with a poor prognosis: a low prothrombin index, marked ascites, GI bleeding, high age, high daily alcohol consumption, high bilirubin, high alkaline phosphatase, low albumin, poor nutritional status and little liver connective tissue inflammation. The last variable, which needs a liver biopsy, can be left out with only little loss of information. Using the pocket chart the prognostic index is not more difficult to calculate than the Child–Turcotte criteria but it provides a better estimate of prognosis. It has been validated using the split sample technique[10]. The index can be translated into an estimate of the probability of surviving the next 3 or 6 months as shown in Figure 1. It is particularly well suited for the follow-up monitoring of patients since it gives a quantitative measure of disease severity and thereby an indication of improvement or deterioration

Table 2 Pocket chart for calculation of current prognostic index in cirrhosis

Variable			*Points to add*
Age (years)	20		0
	30		5
	40		11
	50		16
	60		21
	70		26
	80		31
Current alcohol consumption	none		0
	10–50 g/day		4
	>50 g/day		13
Ascites	none		0
	slight		3
	moderate or marked		12
GI bleeding	no		0
	yes		14
Nutritional status	normal or fat		0
	meagre or cachectic		6
Serum bilirubin	<4 mg/100 ml or <70 μmol/L		0
	≥4 mg/100 ml or ≥70 μmol/L		9
Serum albumin	g/l	μmol/L	
	15	228	–46
	20	304	–50
	30	456	–54
	40	608	–58
	50	760	–61
Prothrombin index (% of normal)	10		22
	15		19
	20		16
	30		13
	40		11
	55		8
	70		6
	105		3
	150		0
Alkaline phosphatase (IU/l)	37		0
	70		2
	107		4
	180		6
	290		8
	400		10
Liver connective tissue inflammation			
	unknown		0
	none or slight		4
	moderate or marked		–2

Sum of points S
Prognostic index PI(t) = S/10 =
Note: For each variable only one number should be used in the addition. If a patient has values between those in the table interpolation should be used.
From Christensen *et al.*[10]

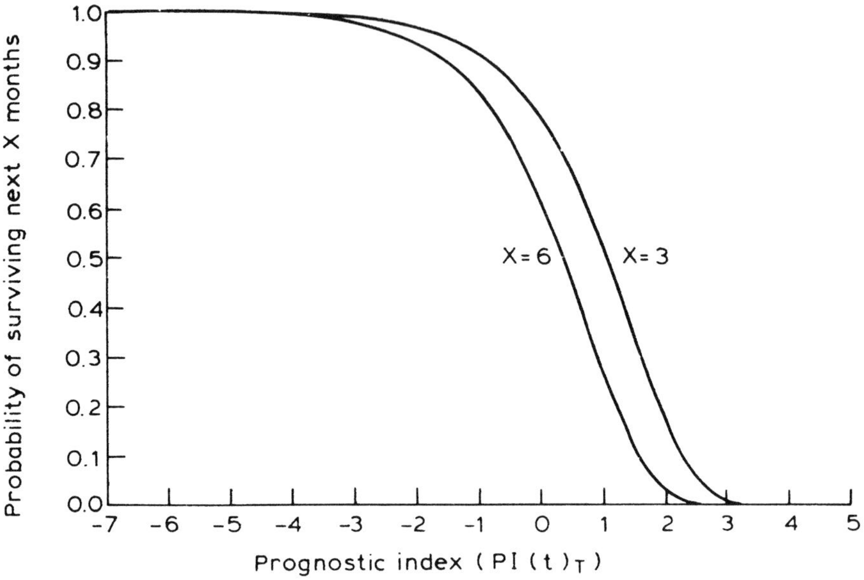

Fig. 1 Estimated probability of surviving the next 3 or 6 months as a function of the current prognostic index in cirrhosis as presented in Table 2. From Christensen *et al.*[10]

during the course of the disease. The index can help in the decision of if and when to perform a liver transplantation in the patient.

The prognostic information of special tests such as the aminopyrine breath test[5,11,12], galactose elimination capacity (GEC)[12], indocyanine green (ICG) intrinsic hepatic clearance[12], plasma noradrenaline[13], portal venous pressure[13,14], and splanchnic angiographic findings[15] have been investigated, but the additional information to that which can be obtained from the clinical variables and simple biochemical tests is generally rather small. The reason for this is that the special tests are to some degree correlated with the clinical variables and the simple biochemical tests which can be obtained easily in the clinical situation. Generally, the simpler the tests and the more easily they can be obtained, the greater the chance that they will achieve general acceptance as prognostic indicators in clinical practice.

ALCOHOLIC LIVER DISEASE

Orrego *et al.* have proposed a combined clinical and laboratory index (CCLI) for global assessment of the severity of alcoholic liver disease[16]. The empirically constructed index was based on 12 variables which in univariate analyses showed significant association with the one-year survival. However, when applying multivariate statistical methods to the data, only 4 of the variables were significantly associated with a poor prognosis (encephalopathy, low albumin, prolonged prothrombin time, low haemoglobin)[16]. The remaining variables seemed to be more or less redundant because of close correlations with the 4 significant ones, showing the value of using multivariate statistical methods for the development of prognostic indices.

Tygstrup *et al.* tested CCLI in independent patients with alcoholic cirrhosis[17]. As might be expected they found a somewhat poorer predictive ability of CCLI than Orrego *et al.* found in their own patients[16]. Using Cox regression analysis, Tygstrup *et al.* found that female gender, high age, low serum acetylcholinesterase activity and ascites were independently associated with a poor prognosis[17].

In 407 patients with alcoholic liver disease included in a large international multicentre trial it was found that a history of alcoholism of long duration, a low prothrombin index, high alkaline phosphatase, high serum creatinine, high immunoglobulin M, high white blood cell count and little liver cell steatosis were all independently associated with a decreased survival[18]. These findings have not yet been validated in independent patients.

CHRONIC HEPATITIS B

Reports on the natural history of chronic hepatitis B are scarce[19,20]. The course of disease is sometimes very long. Therefore surrogate markers such as normalization of alanine aminotransferase (ALT), aspartate aminotransferase (AST), seroconversion (i.e. disappearance of HBeAg, HBsAg and HBV DNA from the serum) have been used in many trials as endpoints for evaluation of therapies including interferon. Within the European concerted action for the study of chronic hepatitis (EUROHEP) a large meta-analysis using individual data from controlled clinical trials including 751 patients demonstrated that interferon increased the HBeAg disappearance rate by a factor of 1.76 during interferon administration[21]. About 3 months after cessation of interferon treatment the HBeAg disappearance rate falls back to the level found during placebo treatment[22]. No information on the effect of interferon on survival or the occurrence of complications is available.

de Jongh *et al.*[20] found, in 98 patients followed up for a mean of 4.3 years, that only age, bilirubin and ascites were independently related to survival. For patients with compensated liver cirrhosis, hepatitis B e antigen (HBeAg) positivity was also a prognostic factor.

Recently a large EUROHEP study on the survival and prognostic factors in 366 patients with chronic hepatitis B and compensated cirrhosis has been performed[23]. The 10-year survival was 68% in these patients. The following variables were found to be associated with a poor prognosis: high age, low albumin, low platelets, splenomegaly, high bilirubin and presence of HBeAg[23]. These variables could be combined into the prognostic index demonstrated in Table 3. This index can be translated into the probability of surviving 5 or 10 years using Figure 2. Although this prognostic score has not been validated using independent data, it may be suited as a surrogate marker for evaluation of treatment effects related to survival. The demonstration of such treatment effects would be a step forward in this disease.

Table 3 Pocket chart for calculation of prognostic index in compensated cirrhosis type B

Variable			*Points to add*
Age (years)	17		6
	28		10
	39		14
	50		18
	61		22
	72		26
	83		30
Serum albumin	g/L	μmol/L	
	20	304	−17
	26	395	−22
	32	486	−27
	38	578	−32
	45	684	−38
	51	775	−43
	57	866	−48
Platelets (× 10^9/L)	35		−2
	85		−5
	135		−8
	205		−12
	270		−16
	340		−20
	405		−24
Splenomegaly	no		0
	yes		5
Serum bilirubin (μmol/L)	14		3
	38		8
	62		13
	86		18
	114		24
	138		29
	162		34
	190		40
HBeAg	no		0
	yes		4

Sum of points S
Prognostic index PI = S/10=
Note: For each variable only one number should be used in the addition. If a patient has values between those in the table, interpolation should be used.
From Realdi *et al.*[23]

CHRONIC HEPATITIS C

Hepatitis C becomes chronic in about 50% of cases but little is known about long-term survival of these patients. Usually the disease progresses very slowly and only after a considerable number of years will cirrhosis and its complications develop. Evaluation of therapies (mainly interferon) has been made using surrogate markers such as normalization of alanine aminotransferase

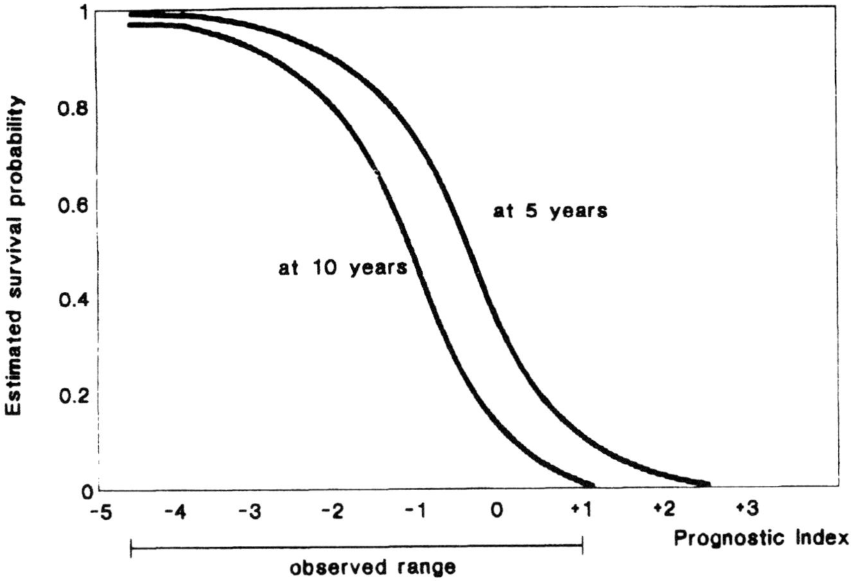

Fig. 2 Estimated probability of surviving 5 or 10 years as a function of the prognostic index in compensated cirrhosis type B as presented in Table 3. From Realdi *et al.*[23]

(ALT), aspartate aminotransferase (AST) and, only recently, disappearance of hepatitis C virus RNA from the serum. Interferon has been shown to have a modest effect on these surrogate markers. The effect of treatments on survival is unknown.

In one multicentre trial[24] the histological activity decreased significantly in responders ($p<0.04$) while the biopsy score did not change significantly in non-responders. In contrast, galactose elimination capacity – a surrogate marker for survival in chronic active hepatitis – was not affected by response to treatment. None of the parameters evaluated, including hepatitis C virus RNA, was able to predict response or relapse.

A large – not yet fully published – EUROHEP study of the natural history of 356 patients with compensated cryptogenic cirrhosis, most of whom have chronic hepatitis C infection, showed that the 10-year survival was 78% for these patients[25]. High age, hepatic stigmata on physical examination, high bilirubin and low platelets were associated with a poor prognosis. These factors can also be combined into a prognostic index which may be a suitable surrogate marker for evaluation of treatment effects related to survival.

PRIMARY BILIARY CIRRHOSIS

Primary biliary cirrhosis is an intrahepatic, chronic, non-suppurative, destructive cholangitis which ultimately leads to cirrhosis. The natural history is one of steady progression but individual courses of disease vary from asymptomatic, with a nearly normal life expectancy, to symptomatic having a more progressive course leading – sooner or later – to liver failure[26]. Many therapies have been tested and although azathioprine, colchicine, methotrexate, cyclosporin A and ursodeoxycholic acid have been reported to have some small beneficial effects[27–30], none of these treatments has been demonstrated effectively to stop progression of the disease. Therefore, in advanced cases liver transplantation is the only effective therapeutic measure.

Since the course of disease is so variable, prognostication in the individual patient becomes important. A number of studies have identified prognostic variables[26,31–38] and devised prognostic indices[32–38]. In 1979 Shapiro demonstrated the paramount importance of serum bilirubin as a prognostic factor[31]. Later a large multinational study of 236 patients identified serum bilirubin, age and histological stage as important independent prognostic variables[26]. In 1983 Roll *et al.* found that elevated bilirubin, old age, hepatomegaly and cirrhosis were associated with a poor prognosis[32]. Using the Cox regression model to analyse the data of an international controlled clinical trial, the following variables were found independently to define a poor prognosis: elevated serum bilirubin, old age, cirrhosis, low serum albumin and central cholestasis[33]. The variables could be combined into a prognostic index which can be calculated for any patient. By applying simple diagrams the calculated prognostic index can be transformed into a probability of surviving a given time or an estimated median survival time[33]. This prognostic index was validated by the demonstration of a good correspondence between the survival predicted by the model and that observed in independent patients divided into 3 groups having a good, medium or poor prognosis[33].

Recently the analyses have been refined to yield a prognostic index for monitoring of patients during the course of the disease[37]. The index utilizes the follow-up information and can be used to update prognosis whenever changes in the condition occur. The index gives more reliable predictions because it is based on a more efficient utilization of data. This monitoring prognostic index is presented as a pocket chart in Table 4. Using the pocket chart it is easy to calculate the prognostic index which can be transformed to probabilities of surviving the next 1, 3 and 6 months using Figure 3. This prognostic index, which has been validated using independent patient data[37], may be particularly useful for optimal timing of liver transplantation.

Other prognostic indices have been proposed in reports from the Mayo Clinic[34], Glasgow[35] and London[36]. The Mayo model comprises age, bilirubin, prothrombin time, albumin and peripheral oedema and exists in two versions, one for prediction of long-term survival[34] and one for prediction of short-term survival[38]. Both versions have been validated using independent patient data[38,39]. The groups from Glasgow[35] and from the Royal Free Hospital in London[36] have devised similar models but these have not yet been validated using independent patients.

Some of the above models have been used to substantiate the value of liver transplantation by demonstrating that the survival observed after the procedure is better than that without, as predicted by the models[40–42]. Such evidence is markedly weaker than that which could have been obtained using controlled clinical trials, but since such have not, and probably will not, be performed, the

Table 4 Pocket chart for calculation of current prognostic index in primary biliary cirrhosis

Variable			*Points to add*
Serum bilirubin	mg/100 ml	μmol/L	
	0.6	10	−6
	1.2	20	1
	2.0	34	7
	2.9	50	11
	4.1	70	15
	5.8	100	19
	8.8	150	23
	11.7	200	27
	17.5	300	31
	23.4	400	34
	29.2	500	37
Ascites	no		0
	yes		14
Serum albumin	g/L	μmol/L	
	20	304	−6
	30	456	−14
	34	517	−18
	40	608	−23
	50	760	−31
	60	912	−40
Age (years)	30		1
	40		5
	50		9
	55		11
	60		13
	70		17
	80		21
GI bleeding	no		0
	yes		7

Sum of points S
Prognostic index PI(t) = S/10 =
Note: For each variable only one number should be used in the addition. If a patient has values between those in the table, interpolation should be used.
From Christensen *et al.*[37]

predictions provided by the prognostic indices have become necessary in the evaluation of the transplantation procedure.

Furthermore, a prognostic model has been devised for prediction of survival after transplantation for primary biliary cirrhosis[43]. Thus it is possible to predict survival time both with and without transplantation and the procedure would accordingly be justified only if the former were longer than the latter.

PRIMARY SCLEROSING CHOLANGITIS

Primary sclerosing cholangitis is a chronic progressive destructive biliary disease of unknown aetiology. The median survival is about 12 years but varies markedly

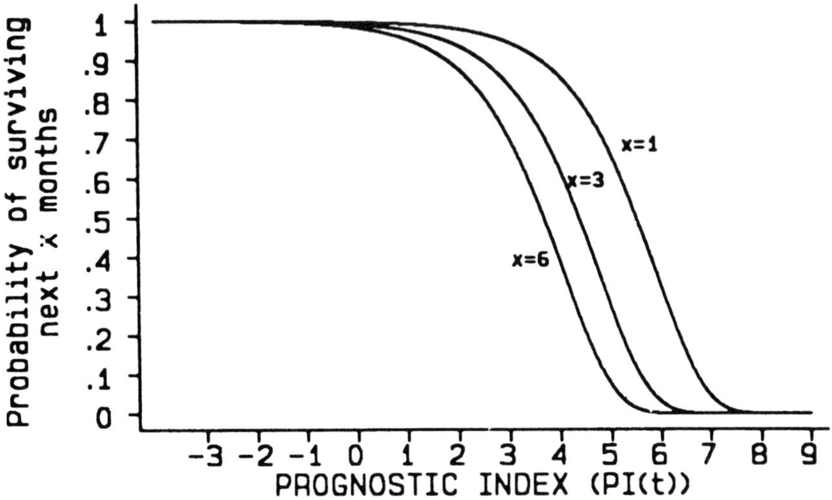

Fig. 3 Estimated probability of surviving the next 1, 3 or 6 months as a function of the current prognostic index in primary biliary cirrhosis as presented in Table 4. From Christensen *et al.*[37]

between individual patients[44–47]. Although minor effects have been reported for ursodeoxycholic acid and methotrexate[48], no medical treatment has been demonstrated effectively to stop progression of the disease. Thus, as with primary biliary cirrhosis, liver transplantation is at present the only effective treatment.

Four prognostic indices have so far been reported[44–47]. Using Cox regression analysis the Mayo Clinic found high age, high bilirubin, low haemoglobin, advanced histological stage and presence of inflammatory bowel disease to be significantly associated with survival[44]. Farrant *et al.* from King's College Hospital found hepatomegaly, splenomegaly, high alkaline phosphatase, advanced histological stage and high age to be independent predictors of a poor prognosis[45]. In a larger study based on 392 patients including both the Mayo and the King's patients, Dickson *et al.* found high bilirubin, high histological stage, high age and splenomegaly to be independent predictors of a poor prognosis[46]. Recently, a large – not yet fully published – Swedish study comprising 305 patients identified high age, high bilirubin and advanced histological stage as independent prognostic indicators[47].

The three first prognostic models have been evaluated in an independent smaller series with regard to the ability to discriminate between patients needing and patients not needing a transplantation[48]. None of the models provided a complete distinction between the two groups but the model of Dickson *et al.*[46] gave the best discrimination[48].

CONCLUSION

Some progress has been made in the development of valid surrogate marker scores which may be suitable for assessing treatments in various chronic liver diseases. A large number of prognostic indices have now been published. Some of these have been validated using independent patient data. Even if the indices are the results of complex statistical analyses, they are not more difficult to use than the Child–Turcotte criteria, because the results can be presented in simple pocket charts and diagrams from which the probability of surviving a given time can be obtained at the bedside.

Nevertheless, there is a need for some simplification and standardization. Within a given disease (e.g. primary biliary cirrhosis) many slightly different prognosis indices have been published. Probably their prognostic information is rather similar, although this has not yet been fully investigated. However, it would be desirable if general agreement could be obtained on one prognostic index to be used as *the* surrogate marker within a given disease. To obtain such an agreement, cooperative studies on combined databases from different centres seem necessary.

The problem in using surrogate markers in the evaluation of treatments should be remembered. One particularly important problem is the following: even if the surrogate marker in untreated patients has been demonstrated to be related to the outcome, it is still possible that the treatment being investigated may influence the surrogate marker *without* having an effect on the course of the disease, i.e. the changes produced by the treatment are purely ‘cosmetic’. The situation will be increasingly complex if the treatment effect varies between individuals[10,49–51] (which may be a more common feature than previously thought) and especially if the variables characterizing responders and non-responders contribute to the surrogate marker index[10,50]. Such problems, which have only been studied sporadically[51], may be much more prominent than we would expect. For these reasons surrogate markers should not be used for evaluation of treatments if hard (or semi-hard) endpoints can be studied. Only if such endpoints cannot be obtained in sufficient numbers within a reasonable time, even in large international multicentre trials, would it be justified to use the surrogate marker scores for treatment evaluation.

References

1. Child CG, Turcotte JG. Surgery and portal hypertension. In Child CG, editor. The liver and portal hypertension. Philadelphia: W.B. Saunders Co., 1964:50.
2. Conn HO. A peek at the Child–Turcotte classification. Hepatology. 1981;1:673–6.
3. Pugh RNH, Murray-Lyon IM, Dawson JL, Pietroni MC, Williams R. Transection of the oesophagus for bleeding oesophageal varices. Br J Surg. 1973;60:646–9.
4. Christensen E, Schlichting P, Fauerholdt L *et al.* Prognostic value of Child–Turcotte criteria in medically treated cirrhosis. Hepatology. 1984;4:430–5.
5. Villeneuve JP, Infante-Rivard C, Ampelas M, Pomier-Layargues G, Huet PM, Marleau D. Prognostic value of the aminopyrine breath test in cirrhotic patients. Hepatology. 1986;6:928–31.
6. Abad Lacruz A, Cabre E, Gonzalez Huix F *et al.* Routine tests of renal function, alcoholism, and nutrition improve the prognostic accuracy of Child–Pugh score in nonbleeding advanced cirrhotics. Am J Gastroenterol. 1993;88:382–7.
7. Schlichting P, Christensen E, Andersen PK *et al.* Prognostic factors in cirrhosis identified by Cox's regression model. Hepatology. 1983;3:889–95.
8. D'Amico G, Morabito A, Pagliaro L, Marubini ETI. Survival and prognostic indicators in compensated and decompensated cirrhosis. Dig Dis Sci. 1986;31:468–75.
9. Gines P, Quintero E, Arroyo V *et al.* Compensated cirrhosis: natural history and prognostic factors. Hepatology. 1987;7:122–8.

10. Christensen E, Schlichting P, Andersen PK *et al.* Updating prognosis and therapeutic effect evaluation in cirrhosis with Cox's multiple regression model for time-dependent variables. Scand J Gastroenterol. 1986;21:163–74.
11. Merkel C, Bolognesi M, Bellon S *et al.* Aminopyrine breath test in the prognostic evaluation of patients with cirrhosis. Gut. 1992;33:836–42.
12. Merkel C, Gatta A, Zoli M *et al.* Prognostic value of galactose elimination capacity, aminopyrine breath test, and ICG clearance in patients with cirrhosis. Comparison with the Pugh score. Dig Dis Sci. 1991;36:1197–203.
13. Tage-Jensen U, Henriksen JH, Christensen E, Widding A, Ring-Larsen H, Christensen NJ. Plasma catecholamine level and portal venous pressure as guides to prognosis in patients with cirrhosis. J Hepatol. 1988;6:350–8.
14. Merkel C, Bolognesi M, Bellon S *et al.* Prognostic usefulness of hepatic vein catheterization in patients with cirrhosis and esophageal varices. Gastroenterology. 1992;102:973–9.
15. Finucci G, Bellon S, Merkel C *et al.* Evaluation of splanchnic angiography as a prognostic index of survival in patients with cirrhosis. Scand J Gastroenterol. 1991;26:951–60.
16. Orrego H, Israel Y, Blake JE *et al.* Assessment of prognostic factors in alcoholic liver disease: Toward a global quantitative expression of severity. Hepatology. 1983;3:896–905.
17. Tygstrup N, Andersen PK, Thomsen BLR. Prognostic evaluation in alcoholic cirrhosis. Acta Med Scand. 1985;Suppl. 703;149–56.
18. Keiding S, Badsberg JH, Becker U *et al.* The prognosis of patients with alcoholic liver disease. An international randomized, placebo-controlled trial on the effect of malothilate on survival. J Hepatol. 1994;20:454–60.
19. Fattovich G, Brollo L, Giustina G *et al.* Natural history and prognostic factors for chronic hepatitis type B. Gut. 1991;32:294–8.
20. de Jongh FE, Janssen HL, de Man RA, Hop WC, Schalm SW, van Blankenstein M. Survival and prognostic indicators in hepatitis B surface antigen-positive cirrhosis of the liver. Gastroenterology. 1992;103:1630–5.
21. Krogsgaard K, Bindslev N, Christensen E *et al.*, and the European concerted action on viral hepatitis (EUROHEP). The treatment effect of alpha interferon in chronic hepatitis B is independent of pre-treatment variables. Results based on individual patient data from 10 clinical controlled trials. J Hepatol. 1994;21:646–55.
22. Krogsgaard K, Christensen E, Bindslev N, Schalm S, Andersen PK, Ring-Larsen H, EUROHEP. The relation between treatment efficacy and the cumulative dose of alfa interferon (IFN) in chronic hepatitis B. (abstract). J Hepatol. 1995;23 suppl. 1:175.
23. Realdi G, Fattovich G, Hadziyannis S *et al.*, and the investigators of the European concerted action on viral hepatitis (EUROHEP). Survival and prognostic factors in 366 patients with compensated cirrhosis type B: a multicenter study. J Hepatol. 1994;21:656–66.
24. Reichen J, Solioz M, Buhler H *et al.* Low-dose interferon in chronic hepatitis non-A/non-B: effects on quantitative liver function and structure in a randomized, controlled multicenter trial. Clin Invest. 1993;71:888–93.
25. Fattowich G, Giustina G, Degos F *et al.*, EUROHEP EPIDEMIOLOGY. Survival and prognostic indicators in cryptogenic compensated cirrhosis: A multicenter study. (abstract). J Hepatol. 1995;23 suppl. 1:122.
26. Christensen E, Crowe J, Doniach D *et al.* Clinical pattern and course of disease in primary biliary cirrhosis based on an analysis of 236 patients. Gastroenterology. 1980;78:236–46.
27. Wiesner RH, Grambsch PM, Lindor KD *et al.* Clinical and statistical analysis of new and evolving therapies for primary biliary cirrhosis. Hepatology. 1988;8:668–76.
28. Slitzky BE, Quellette GS, Boyer JL. Approaches to the treatment of primary biliary cirrhosis – A status report. Gastroenterol Int. 1990;3:134–9.
29. Lombard M, Portmann B, Neuberger J *et al.* Cyclosporin A treatment in primary biliary cirrhosis. Results of a long-term placebo controlled trial. Gastroenterology. 1993;104:519–26.
30. Leuschner U. Ursodeoxycholic acid therapy in primary biliary cirrhosis. Scand J Gastroenterol. 1994;29 suppl. 204:40–6.
31. Shapiro JM, Smith H, Schaffner F. Serum bilirubin: a prognostic factor in primary biliary cirrhosis. Gut. 1979;20:137–40.
32. Roll J, Boyer JL, Barry D, Klatskin G. The prognostic importance of clinical and histologic features in asymptomatic and symptomatic primary biliary cirrhosis. N Engl J Med. 1983;308:1–7.

33. Christensen E, Neuberger J, Crowe J *et al.* Beneficial effect of azathioprine and prediction of prognosis in primary biliary cirrhosis. Final results of an international trial. Gastroenterology. 1985;89:1084–91.
34. Dickson ER, Grambsch PM, Fleming TR, Fisher LD, Langworthy A. Prognosis in primary biliary cirrhosis: a model for decision making. Hepatology. 1989;10:1–7 .
35. Goudie BM, Burt AD, Macfarlane GJ *et al.* Risk factors and prognosis in primary biliary cirrhosis. Am J Gastroenterol. 1989;84:713–6.
36. Hughes MD, Raskino CL, Pocock SJ, Biagini MR, Burroughs AK. Prediction of short-term survival with an application in primary biliary cirrhosis. Stat Med. 1992;11:1731–45.
37. Christensen E, Altman DG, Neuberger J, De Stavola BL, Tygstrup N, Williams R, PBC1 and PBC2 trial groups. Updating prognosis in primary biliary cirrhosis using a time-dependent Cox regression model. Gastroenterology. 1993;105:1865–76.
38. Murtaugh PA, Dickson ER, Van Dam GM *et al.* Primary biliary cirrhosis: prediction of short-term survival based on repeated patient visits. Hepatology. 1994;20:126–34.
39. Jeffrey GP, Hoffman NE, Reed WD. Validation of prognostic models in primary biliary cirrhosis. Aus NZ J Med. 1990;20:107–10.
40. Neuberger J, Altman DG, Christensen E, Tygstrup N, Williams R. Use of a prognotic index in evaluation of liver transplantation for primary biliary cirrhosis. Transplantation. 1986;41:713–6.
41. Markus B, Dickson ER, Grambsch PM *et al.* Efficacy of liver transplantation in patients with primary biliary cirrhosis. N Engl J Med. 1989;320:1709–13.
42. Bonsel GJ, Klompmaker IJ, van't Veer F, Habbema JD, Slooff MJ. Use of prognostic models for assessment of value of liver transplantation in primary biliary cirrhosis. Lancet. 1990;335:493–7.
43. Neuberger J, Altman DG, Polson R *et al.* Prognosis after liver transplantation for primary biliary cirrhosis. Transplantation. 1989;48:444–7.
44. Wiesner RH, Grambsch PM, Dickson ER *et al.* Primary sclerosing cholangitis: natural history, prognostic factors and survival analysis. Hepatology. 1989;10:430–6.
45. Farrant JM, Hayllar KM, Wilkinson ML *et al.* Natural history and prognostic variables in primary sclerosing cholangitis. Gastroenterology. 1991;100:1710–7.
46. Dickson ER, Murtaugh PA, Wiesner RH *et al.* Primary sclerosing cholangitis: refinement and validation of survival models. Gastroenterology. 1992;103:1136–41.
47. Broome U, Olofsson L, Loof L *et al.* Natural history and prognostic factors in 305 Swedish patients with primary sclerosing cholangitis. (abstract). J Hepatol. 1995;23 suppl. 1:166.
48. Broome U, Eriksson LS. Assessment for liver transplantation in patients with primary sclerosing cholangitis. J Hepatol. 1994;20:654–9.
49. Copenhagen Study Group for Liver Diseases. Sex, ascites and alcoholism in survival of patients with cirrhosis. Effect of prednisone. N Engl J Med. 1974;291:271–3.
50. Christensen E, Schlichting P, Andersen PK *et al.* A therapeutic index that predicts the individual effect of prednisone in patients with cirrhosis. Gastroenterology. 1985;88:156–65.
51. Christensen E. Individual therapy-dependent prognosis based on data from controlled clinical trials in chronic liver disease. Dan Med Bull. 1988;35:167–82.

7
Validation of surrogate markers for death in cirrhosis: an example using decrease in galactose elimination capacity

C. MERKEL, G. MARCHESINI, A. FABBRI, S. BIANCO, G. BIANCHI, E. ENZO, A. GATTA and E. PISI

INTRODUCTION

A surrogate endpoint is an endpoint which is used to define effectiveness of a treatment instead of the clinically relevant endpoint, because either the real one is too remote to be waited for, too expensive or too difficult to be measured. The term surrogate does not imply a negative denotation, but only reflects the use as a substitute (from the Latin *surrogare* = to substitute). The use of surrogate endpoints was developed in order to limit the cost and the time needed to reach a conclusion in clinical trials. The interpretation of trials based on surrogate endpoints may be difficult, and serious controversies arose in recent years when the direct relation between surrogate and real endpoint was doubtful. For instance, the Food and Drug Administration in 1987 did not accept arterial clot dissolution as a surrogate for cardiovascular mortality in a trial of thrombolytic therapy, and tumour response rate as a surrogate for total mortality in the treatment of breast cancer[1]. Indeed, in all these cases, the surrogate endpoint was related to the true endpoint, but did not take into account the rate of complications.

Before a surrogate endpoint can be used in clinical practice, its suitability must first be shown in the clinical situation under study, and with the therapeutic options under study. Indeed, a suitable surrogate endpoint for one treatment may be unsuitable for another treatment, if the first treatment only influences the occurrence of the true endpoint via mechanism(s) related to the occurrence of the surrogate endpoint, and the second treatment does not. For instance, occurrences of ascites may be a reasonable surrogate endpoint for liver related mortality in cirrhosis, but only if the treatment under study itself has no direct influence on the sodium balance.

A more stringent method of validating a surrogate endpoint is to analyse a trial or a series of trials performed on the clinical problem under study, to verify if (or to what extent) a surrogate endpoint meets the criteria proposed by Prentice[2]. In particular, the first criterion requires that the occurrence of the surrogate endpoint is linked to the occurrence of the true endpoint; the second criterion requires that the mechanism(s) through which treatment influences the true endpoint involves directly and concurrently the occurrence of the surrogate one.

Preliminary data have suggested a possible use of quantitative liver function test (QLFT) variations as surrogate markers for survival in patients with chronic liver disease[3]. The first Prentice criterion is proven by the strict association of decrease in QLFT and survival shown in many series[4–6]. Compliance with the second criterion is more difficult to prove, since it should be done for every single treatment to be analysed. From a practical point of view, the current lack of treatments which consistently improve liver function and consequently survival in chronic liver disease, makes this problem a theoretical one at the present time. However, abstinence from alcohol in alcoholic cirrhosis may be considered a model for a drug treatment improving survival through improvement in liver function, and the different course of values of a QLFT in patients who start abstinence, compared to that of patients who continue drinking, may mimic the effect of a drug treatment in a clinical trial.

As an example of the methods of validation, in this preliminary analysis we assessed the possible use of decrease in galactose elimination capacity (GEC) as a possible marker for death in cirrhotics with alcohol abuse, trying to validate compliance with the second criterion. If improvement in GEC in patients who start abstinence is strictly linked to increase in survival, this will be a clue to the possible use of GEC as a surrogate marker for survival in this disease under this treatment.

AN EXAMPLE

Forty-three cirrhotic patients with chronic alcohol abuse were retrospectively selected from patients followed with GEC determinations at six-month intervals in the Departments of Medicine of the Universities of Bologna and Padua. Patients were divided into a group of persistent drinkers (21 patients, group A) and a group of persistent abstainers (22 patients, group B).

To assess the possible value of decrease in GEC as surrogate marker for liver-related death, the method proposed by Lin *et al.*[7] was used. For this purpose, a series of Cox regression models[8] were built. First, separate models for alcohol abuse and for decrease in GEC were built, considering GEC as a time-dependent variable. Then, changes in significance of alcohol abuse were analysed when GEC was added as a time-dependent variable to alcohol abuse itself. According to this analysis, if alcohol abuse loses its value as a predictor of death when GEC is added, GEC is capturing most of the prognostic value of alcohol abuse, and alcohol abuse therefore influences survival through its effect on GEC.

During follow-up 10 patients in group A and 3 patients in group B died from liver-related causes. Persistent alcohol abuse was significantly related to survival

Table 1 Cox's regression model for the 43 patients with cirrhosis

Model	*Variable*	*β*	*β/SEM*	*p*
Only alcohol abuse				
	Abuse	0.62	2.09	0.04
Only GEC (time-dependent)				
	GEC	–1.05	–3.97	0.01
Alcohol abuse and GEC (time-dependent)				
	GEC	–0.97	–3.47	0.01
	Abuse	0.32	0.97	0.33

according to Cox's regression analysis. GEC was also significantly related to survival according to a time-dependent Cox regression analysis (Table 1). When a Cox's model containing time-dependent GEC values and alcohol abuse was built, GEC turned out to be strictly related to survival, while alcohol abuse was no longer significant (Table 1). The present Cox's regression analysis implies that risk of death for persistent alcohol abuse was approximately 3.5 times higher than that of patients who abstained, and that risk of death increased by 34% for every decrease of GEC by 1 mg/kg/min. Although persistent alcohol abuse and decrease in GEC were both significant predictors of death, they were not statistically independent, i.e. they were not expressions of different mechanisms leading to death. In fact, decrease in GEC incorporated most of the prognostic information from persistent alcohol abuse, and a 2-variable model showed that persistent alcohol abuse was no longer significant when variations in GEC were taken into account.

This implies that variations in risk of death occurring as a consequence of abstinence from alcohol may be predicted from changes in GEC, and that the mechanisms through which abstinences influence survival are strictly linked to the mechanisms which cause changes in GEC. This represents adherence to the second criterion proposed by Prentice[2]. Taken together with the strict association of decrease in GEC and survival[5, 6], this observation suggests that GEC may be a useful surrogate endpoint for survival in this clinical condition. When new therapies aiming at improving survival in cirrhosis by improving liver function or delaying the progressive decrease of liver function are available, the use of GEC decrease as a surrogate marker will be worth testing.

References

1. Herson J. The use of surrogate endpoints in clinical trials (an introduction to a series of four papers). Stat Med. 1989;8:403–4.
2. Prentice RL. Surrogate endpoints in clinical trials: Definitions and operational criteria. Stat Med. 1989;8:431–40.
3. Reichen J, Solioz M, Buehler H *et al.* Low-dose interferon in chronic hepatitis non-A/non-B: Effect on quantitative liver function and structure in a randomized controlled multicenter trial. Clin Invest. 1993;71:888–93.
4. Merkel C, Bolognesi M, Bellon S *et al.* Aminopyrine breath test in the prognostic evaluation of patients with cirrhosis. Gut. 1992;33:836–42.
5. Merkel C, Gatta A, Zoli M *et al.* Prognostic value of galactose elimination capacity, aminopyrine breath test, and ICG clearance in patients with cirrhosis. Comparison with the Pugh score. Dig Dis Sci. 1991;36:1197–203.

6. Reichen J, Widmer T, Cotting J. Accurate prediction of death by serial determinations of galactose elimination capacity in primary biliary cirrhosis: A comparison with the Mayo model. Hepatology. 1991;14:504–10.
7. Lin DY, Fischl MA, Schoenfeld DA. Evaluation the role of CD4-lymphocyte count as surrogate endpoints in human immunodeficiency virus clinical trials. Stat Med. 1993;12:835–42.
8. Cox DR. Regression models and life tables (with discussion). J R Stat Soc. 1972;B34:187–220.

8
Quantitative liver function tests as surrogate markers for end points in controlled clinical trials

E. LOTTERER, J. HÖGEL, W. GAUS, W. E. FLEIG and J. BIRCHER

Quantitative liver function tests such as the determination of galactose elimination capacity (GEC) or the aminopyrine breath test (ABT) may have the potential to serve as refined entry criteria and surrogate markers for endpoints in controlled clinical trials. The magnitude of a statistically significant difference in test results and the period of observation required to document such a difference must be known in order to design such trials properly. Therefore, we explored retrospectively the time course of changes in GEC and ABT and their reproducibility from a cohort of patients with alcoholic cirrhosis followed for 32 months (median; range: 12–42 months). In 15 patients who stopped drinking, GEC improved significantly from 3.0 mg/min/kg (1.5–4.9) to 4.0 mg/min/kg (2.5–6.1; $p<0.01$). In contrast, it deteriorated from 4.8 mg/min/kg (3.3–5.8) to 3.0 mg/min/kg (2.1–5.2; $p<0.01$) in another 17 patients who continued to drink. The standard deviation of the test and the corresponding 95%-confidence interval was 0.46 (0.37–0.61) mg/min/kg. In addition, ABT improved significantly from 0.16%dose × kg/mmolCO_2 (0.01–0.49) to 0.40%dose × kg/mmolCO_2 (0.15–0.74; $p<0.01$) in the abstinent group and deteriorated from 0.25% dose × kg/mmolCO_2 (0.04–0.76) to 0.10%dose × kg/mmolCO_2 (0.02–0.48; $p<0.05$) in the non-abstinent group. The standard deviation of the ABT and the corresponding 95%-confidence interval was 0.08 (0.06–0.11)% dose × kg/ mmolCO_2.

As calculated from these data, treatments to be tested in clinical trials with a sample size of $n=20$ in each group must achieve absolute differences in GEC of 0.6 mg/min/kg and of 0.8 mg/min/kg to reach statistical significance at the 5% and 1% level, respectively. In the present study a period of 12 and 14 months was necessary to observe such differences. The corresponding results for the ABT are 0.12%dose × kg/mmolCO_2 (10 months follow-up) and 0.14% dose × kg/ mmolCO_2 (12 months observation), respectively. Provided that patients with liver diseases treated with drugs behave similar to the abstinent and non-abstinent patients with alcoholic liver disease investigated in this study, such numbers could serve for the planning of controlled clinical trials, in which the control group is likely to deteriorate and the treated group is expected to improve. Trials based on GEC or ABT would require only 40 or 34 patient-years of observation compared to the 50 to 2100 patient-years reported for various published controlled clinical trials using survival analysis.

Section III
Cirrhosis and Portal Hypertension

9
The Child–Turcotte and Child–Pugh classifications

N. McINTYRE

Patients with cirrhosis may suffer serious complications, the treatment of which is potentially hazardous. Not surprisingly efforts have been made to determine the prognosis of the cirrhosis *per se*, and the likely outcome of therapeutic intervention. But if a classification of the severity of liver disease is to be widely used it must be simple, practical and relatively cheap, i.e. based on clinical criteria which can be easily assessed, and on the results of tests available in many laboratories.

In 1964 Child and Turcotte described a simple system of grading patients with cirrhosis (Table 1) to assess 'the liver's capacity to withstand not only the strain of operation [for portal decompression] but also the substantial ravages of hemorrhage, ascites and hypersplenism'[1]. It was virtually identical to a classification presented three years earlier by Wantz and Payne[2], but it became known as the Child–Turcotte system, or simply Child's system (even Turcotte used this name in 1973). The authors considered it to be based upon hepatic functional reserve. It took account of the serum bilirubin and albumin levels, the nutritional state and the absence or severity of ascites and encephalopathy. Patients were allocated to group A (good hepatic function), B (moderately impaired hepatic function) or C (advanced hepatic dysfunction). Encephalopathy was considered the least useful criterion by Child and Turcotte. The choice of criteria was

Table 1 Child's grading of the severity of liver disease

Clinical and biochemical measurements	*Child's grade*		
	A	*B*	*C*
Bilirubin (mg/100 ml)	<2.0	2.0–3.0	>3.0
Albumin (g/L)	>35	30–35	<30
Ascites	Absent controlled	Easily controlled	Poorly
Encephalopathy	None	Minimal	Advanced, 'coma'
Nutrition	Excellent	Good	Poor, 'wasting'

arbitrary, but clearly based on clinical experience. It is of interest that although we still do not fully understand the factors causing encephalopathy, ascites and malnutrition in patients with cirrhosis, we recognize that these conditions are good evidence of hepatic 'decompensation'.

There are several problems with the Child–Turcotte system. The main one is that the authors gave no clear guidelines for its use. They seemed to imply that a patient allocated to group A, B or C group would exhibit all of the criteria characterizing that group. Certainly they did not state whether allocation to group B or C should be made if only one of the relevant criteria was present; this was unfortunate as many patients with cirrhosis show a mixture of features from columns A, B and C in Table 1. As Conn[3] pointed out, if patients are categorized as A or C only if they have a 'full house' of the appropriate findings, there will be an excess of grade B patients. If only one criterion is needed there will be an excess in group C. Different groups have applied the Child–Turcotte criteria in different ways. For example, Cello *et al.*[4] designated patients as Child's C on the basis of the single worst criterion for class C, while for Warren *et al.*[5], two or more of these criteria were needed for the same purpose.

In an attempt to resolve this difficulty Lord *et al.*[6] and Campbell and Parker[7] assigned a number to the five criteria originally proposed by Wantz and Payne, and subsequently by Child and Turcotte, designating an A criterion as 1, a B as 2, and C as 3; they added the five scores to obtain a total score ranging from 5–15. This approach removed one ambiguity inherent in the Child–Turcotte system. However, Lord *et al.* categorized a patient as grade A when the score was 5–7, B when it was 8–12, and grade C when it was 13–15; Campbell *et al.* used the total scores 5–8, 9–11, and 12–15 for these grades. The choice of total scores for grading has important implications (see later).

The other main problem is that disagreement between observers is inevitable if they have to decide whether ascites is 'easily' or 'poorly' controlled, neurological disorder 'minimal' or 'advanced', or nutritional status 'excellent' or just 'good' (most workers using the Child–Turcotte method changed the nutritional criteria!).

The grading system which now appears to be more widely used is that of Pugh *et al.*[8], often called the Child–Pugh system, which was introduced to assess operative risk in patients undergoing surgical transection of the oesophagus for variceal bleeding (Table 2). These authors used the same point scoring system as

Table 2 Pugh's grading of the severity of liver disease

Clinical and biochemical measurements	*Points scored for increasing abnormality*		
	1	*2*	*3*
Encephalopathy[a]	None	1 and 2	3 and 4
Ascites	Absent	Slight	Moderate
Bilirubin (mg/100 ml)	1–2	2–3	>3
Albumin (g/L)	>35	28–35	<28
Prothrombin (s prolonged)	1–4	4–6	>6
For primary biliary cirrhosis			
Bilirubin (mg/100 ml)	1–4	4–10	>10

[a] According to grading of Trey *et al.*[9]

Lord *et al.* and Campbell *et al.*, but a total score of 5–6 led to allocation to group A, 7–9 to group B, and 10–15 to C. They adjusted the score allocated for the bilirubin level in primary biliary cirrhosis, as the level of bilirubin in this condition is often out of proportion to other evidence of hepatic failure; Wantz and Payne, and Child and Turcotte, also realized the need for this adjustment. As D'Heygere and Burroughs[10] pointed out, this modification is clinically appropriate, but in the emergency situation it does presume that the correct diagnosis is known at the time of assessing the patient.

There were some minor differences from the Child–Turcotte system in Pugh's classification. The grading system of Trey *et al.*[9] was used to allocate the score for encephalopathy; there was a slight change in the albumin level used to differentiate between a score of 2 and 3 (28 instead of 30 g/L, although most workers seem to have used 30 g/L even when they claimed to use Pugh's method); and the terms 'absent', 'slight' and 'moderate' were used to assess ascites (this remains an ambiguous component, particularly as some groups have used ultrasonography rather than clinical examination to determine the absence of ascites). However, the main difference was that Pugh's system included the prothrombin time and dispensed with nutritional status. The authors gave no reason for these changes, and there was no statistical basis for the classification. In the paper little attention was paid to the grading system. According to Westaby[11] it was invented over lunch one day by a medical intern, on the basis of a discussion between experienced surgeons and physicians.

The switch from nutritional status to prothrombin time was sensible. Many studies attest to the value of the prothrombin time in assessing prognosis (in acute and chronic liver disease), although the INR should probably be substituted for the prothrombin time[10]. However, many clinicians still consider nutritional status to be an important prognostic factor in cirrhosis. Unfortunately it is relatively difficult to assess in simple terms. Anthropometric measures are certainly valuable for quantifying changes in nutritional status, but they are unsatisfactory for assessing it at a single time point in an individual patient, unless the results fall well outside the wide normal ranges. Other nutritional measures are even more difficult to apply in routine practice. Even so it is likely that most clinicians regard patients as being a poor risk when they are obviously malnourished (as is evident from the original wording in the Child–Turcotte criteria).

The Child–Turcotte and Pugh systems are relatively crude methods of assessment. Initially they were used to assess prognosis in patients who were candidates for surgical (and later) endoscopic therapy of variceal bleeding and portal hypertension, either electively or as an emergency. They both serve well for this purpose. Grade A patients tend to do well; grade C patients do poorly; the results in grade B patients fall in between, but are usually closer to the results in grade A patients[3]; an example of the sort of results obtained is presented in Figure 1. This was hardly a surprising finding. All experienced hepatologists realize that jaundiced patients with a low albumin, and with ascites encephalopathy and/or poor nutritional status (or a prolonged prothrombin time) have a poor outlook, and that those without these features do well.

Child's grading has also been found useful for assessing the prognosis of other surgical procedures in cirrhotics. In patients treated surgically for gall-

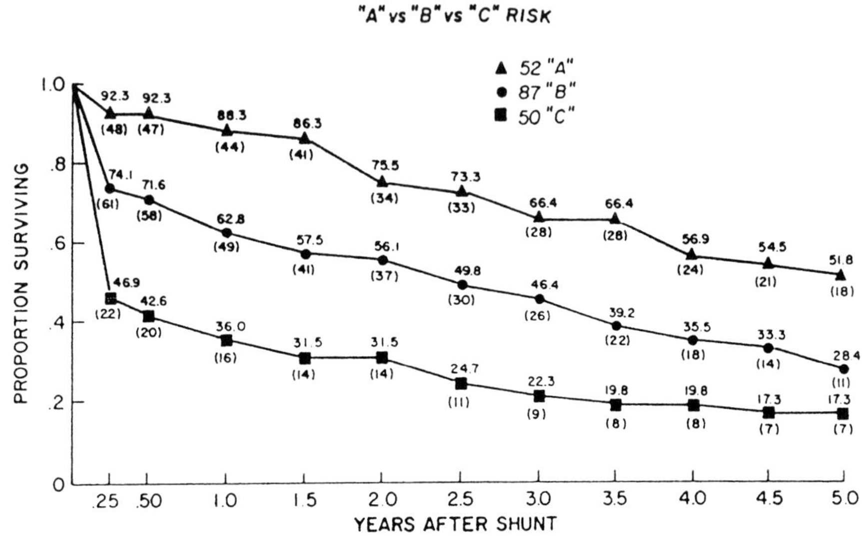

Fig. 1 Cumulative survival of patients undergoing portacaval operations based on hepatic risk class. These survival estimates include all patients who die within the first three months of operation. The numbers above the lines are the probability of survival to the various intervals. The numbers below the lines are the numbers of patients available for observation at the beginning of each interval (from reference 12 with permission)

stones the mortality was much higher in Child's grade C patients than in those who were grades A and B; indeed in two studies there was little or no mortality in grade A and B patients for either emergency or elective procedures[13,14]. Garrison *et al.*[15] found a striking relationship between mortality and Child's grading for all types of intra-abdominal procedure in cirrhotic patients. These results indicate the need for great caution before embarking on surgery in grade C patients.

It is hardly surprising that physicians have used the Child–Turcotte and Pugh–Child criteria to assess prognosis in non-surgical patients. Again the relationship between mortality and Child's status has been confirmed. Two recent studies illustrate this point. Mondazzi *et al.*[16] used transarterial oily chemoembolization to treat patients with hepatocellular carcinoma. They excluded Child–Pugh C patients, but found a significantly higher mortality in grade B patients than in grade A; as one might expect they also found a number of other factors to be of prognostic significance, e.g. age, tumour size and change in alpha-fetoprotein concentration. Bernard *et al.*[17] studied bacterial infection in bleeding cirrhotic patients. The Child–Pugh score was significantly higher in those who became infected, and the risk of rebleeding was significantly linked to the Child–Pugh score. More importantly, in their multivariate analysis only the Child–Pugh score was predictive of death.

In view of the arbitrary way in which the Child–Turcotte and Child–Pugh systems seem to have originated it was to be expected that a better method of prognostic classification would be sought. There are, of course, major problems in deciding on the prognostic value of variables which appear to be useful on the basis of a retrospective analysis, as it is necessary to test them on a new population of patients to assess their prognostic validity. Many workers fail to take this into account.

Campbell and Parker[7] failed to find a better method. They considered Child's original criteria (but used with a 1–3 scoring system) to be 'as good a set of easily obtained predictive parameters as is presently available'. Smith *et al.*[18] correlated 21 variables with immediate and long-term postoperative morbidity (in patients with portal hypertension treated with interposition shunts) and confirmed, 'once again, the value of the Child's criteria in the assessment of the cirrhotic patient.'

In 1984 Christensen *et al.*[19] published a detailed evaluation of the prognostic value of the original Child–Turcotte criteria applied to cirrhotic patients treated medically over a long period of time. They used the 1–3 scoring system employed by Lord *et al.*[6], Campbell and Parker[7], and Pugh *et al.*[8], but their choice of total scores for allocation to grades A (5–7), B (8–10) and C (11–15) was different to that chosen by the other three groups. They compared the value of the Child–Turcotte score with that of 36 other prognostic variables.

Unfortunately, because of their method of selection, 70% of their patients were grade A and only 6% grade C. They found a statistically significant trend of decreasing survival time with increasing total score, and felt that the use of the total score markedly increased the prognostic information when compared with a simple classification into grades A, B and C. Although they recognized that the Child–Turcotte criteria may be useful for a quick assessment of prognosis, because they are simple and easily applicable in clinical practice, they concluded that the prognostic value of the Child–Turcotte criteria is incomplete, and suggested that other variables have additional prognostic information[20]. A number of the other variables which they proposed are, however, impractical for use in clinical practice.

Infante-Rivard *et al.*[21] considered the simplicity of the Child–Turcotte classification to be important and that this point had not been given sufficient weight. They evaluated it with regard to short-term (1-year) survival in 177 cirrhotic patients, but they employed the Child–Pugh modification. Their analysis was a complicated one, but they found that classification into grades A, B and C captured less variance than the Pugh score counted from 5 to 15, which in turn captured less variance than a mathematical model in which indices of Pugh score were analysed according to their original units. As the 5–15 score was almost as good as the mathematical model they suggested that the total score was satisfactory for routine clinical practice. They also suggested that the qualities of simplicity, availability, low cost and good discriminating power for a life or death outcome make the Pugh score a very useful method to estimate prognosis in patients with cirrhosis, and that it should be used as a standard of reference when evaluating new prognostic tests or models.

From the work of Christensen *et al.*[19] and Infante- Rivard *et al.*[21] it might seem sensible to use the total score (5–15) rather than classification into groups A, B and C when assessing prognosis, but this approach, which would result in 11 groups, would be of limited value unless a trial involved large numbers of patients.

In a simpler study Albers *et al.*[22] compared the prognostic value of the Child–Pugh classification with that of 15 other variables, including galactose elimination capacity and indocyanine green clearance. They used a Kaplan–Meier life-table analysis and Cox proportional hazards regression analysis to analyse data obtained from 47 patients with cirrhosis. They found the Child–Pugh grade to be the best predictive factor of survival over several years.

Even though the Child–Turcotte and Child–Pugh systems are relatively simple to use, I suspect that few of us bother to allocate patients formally to grades A, B or C for the purposes of management, although we almost certainly take the Child–Turcotte criteria and the prothrombin time (or INR) into account when deciding about the risks of treatment. But we also have to consider many other factors when making our decisions, including portal hypertension and variceal bleeding, renal dysfunction, nutritional status, and cardiovascular and respiratory disorders.

The importance of grading comes when one is trying to assess the value of different forms of therapy. This requires comparisons of outcome to be made in relatively large groups of patients. For this purpose it is essential that the classification of groups should be based on the same criteria. Logic dictates that if an inappropriately large number of patients are allocated to group C (e.g. by lowering the total score required for classification as group C, or by demanding only one grade C criterion) patients will be shifted from group B to group C, and that one would then expect a better outcome both in group C and in group B. There would be a similar improvement in both groups if patients who should be allocated to group A are transferred to group B. This is evident in the paper of D'Heygere and Burroughs[10] in which they presented results from the same group of patients but classified using the methods of Campbell and Parker, Pugh *et al.* and Cello *et al.* (Table 3). Further support for this proposition can be found in the paper by Conn[3], reviewing nine different studies, in which there seems to be an inverse relationship between the proportion of patients allocated to group C and the mortality after shunt surgery (Figure 2); the proposition could also explain the difference in mortality rates for other types of abdominal surgery in the papers of Bloch *et al.*[13] and Garrison *et al.*[15].

Table 3 Comparison of modified Child's classification in a consecutive series of cirrhotics admitted with variceal bleeding at the Royal Free Hospital (from reference 10)

	Grade		
	A	*B*	*C*
Number of patients: 132			
Campbell	42%	37%	21%
Pugh	20%	36%	45%
Cello	6%	28%	66%
Number of deaths: 30			
Campbell	7%	23%	52%
Pugh	4%	13%	37%
Cello	13%	5%	30%

(D'Heygere and Burroughs, 1987[10])

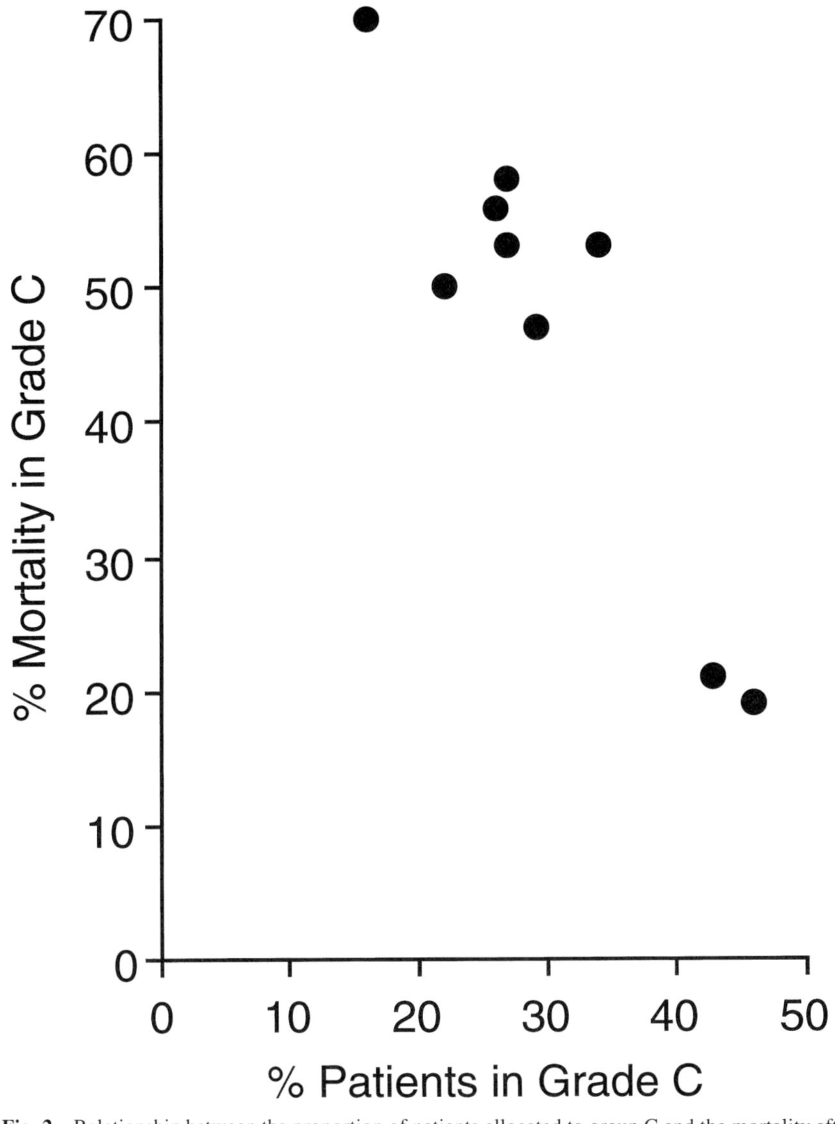

Fig. 2 Relationship between the proportion of patients allocated to group C and the mortality after shunt surgery (date adapted from reference 3)

There are two issues which have received little or no attention when the prognostic significance of the Child–Turcotte and Child–Pugh systems is evaluated. One is that gradings are usually done at one point in time. When surgery or sclerotherapy is to be carried out the time chosen is usually just before the procedure is carried out. The grading may then be influenced by extrinsic factors;

e.g. the bilirubin may be higher because of recent transfusion, encephalopathy may be worse due to medication, and ascites may appear because of inadvertent fluid overload. To the best of my knowledge no one has checked whether patients who have been persistently grade C do worse than those who have been tipped from grade A or B into grade C as a result of recent events. One might expect the latter group to have a better prognosis with the potential of returning to their original grade. Five of the 13 Child's C patients discharged by Cello *et al.*[4] following sclerotherapy for bleeding varices subsequently improved their Child's status (but note that these authors designated patients as Child's C on the basis of the single worst criterion for Class C).

The other issue is whether one can legitimately claim to improve the grade, and thus the prognosis, by treating ascites or encephalopathy, or by increasing the serum albumin by infusing large amounts of albumin. Spontaneous improvement in these indices should clearly be accepted for the purposes of reclassification.

On the basis of current evidence we believe that the Child–Pugh system is probably the best method of assessing the short-term prognosis in patients with cirrhosis. The longer-term prognosis is more likely to be influenced by factors such as abstention from alcohol, or specific therapy for individual diseases. It seems unlikely that a simpler method of assessment will be found, and more detailed classifications are unlikely to find favour in clinical practice. However, it would be beneficial if all clinicians used the Child–Pugh system in the same way, and it would help if clear guidelines could be agreed for allocating the scores for ascites and encephalopathy.

References

1. Child CG, Turcotte JG. Surgery and portal hypertension. In: Child CG, editor. The liver and portal hypertension, Volume 1 in Major Problems of Surgery Series. Philadelphia: Saunders, 1964.
2. Wantz GE, Payne MA. Experience with portacaval shunt for portal hypertension. N Engl J Med. 1961;265:721–8.
3. Conn HO. A peek at the Child–Turcotte classification. Hepatology. 1981;1:673–6.
4. Cello JP, Grendell JH, Crass RA *et al.* Endoscopic sclerotherapy versus porta-caval shunt in patients with severe cirrhosis and variceal haemorrhage. N Engl J Med. 1984;311:1589–94.
5. Warren WD, Henderson JM, Millikan WJ *et al.* Distal splenorenal shunt versus endoscopic sclerotherapy for long-term management of variceal bleeding. Ann Surg. 1986;203:454–61.
6. Lord JW, Rossi G, Daliana M, Rosati LM. Portsystemic shunts in the management of massive haemorrhage from esophageal varices due to cirrhosis of the liver. Am J Surg. 1971;121:241–8.
7. Campbell DP, Parker DE, Anagnostopoulos CE. Survival prediction in portacaval shunts: a computerized statistical analysis. Am J Surg. 1973;126:748–51.
8. Pugh RNH, Murray-Lyon IM, Dawson JL, Pietroni MC, Williams R. Transection of the oesophagus for bleeding oesophageal varices. Br J Surg. 1973;60:646–9.
9. Trey C, Burns DG, Saunders SJ. Treatment of hepatic coma by exchange blood transfusions. N Engl J Med. 1966;274:473–81.
10. D'Heygere F, Burroughs AK. Classification of patients. In: Burroughs AK, editor. Methodology and reviews of clinical trials in portal hypertension, Excerpta Medica International Congress Series No. 763. 1987:41–8.
11. Westaby D. In: Burroughs AK, editor. Methodology and reviews of clinical trials in portal hypertension, Excerpta Medica International Congress Series No. 763. 1987:50.
12. Turcotte JG, Lambert MJ. Variceal hemorrhage, hepatic cirrhosis and portacaval shunts. Surgery. 1973;73:810–7.

13. Bloch RS, Allaben RD, Walt AJ. Cholecystectomy in patients with cirrhosis. A surgical challenge. Arch Surg. 1985;120:669–72.
14. Wu CC, Hwang CJ, Liu TJ. Definitive surgical treatment of cholelithiasis in selective patients with liver cirrhosis. Int Surg. 1993;78:127–30.
15. Garrison RN, Cryer HM, Howard DA, Polk HC. Clarification of risk factors for abdominal operations in patients with hepatic cirrhosis. Ann Surg. 1984;199:648–55.
16. Mondazzi L, Bottelli R, Brambilla G *et al.* Transarterial oily chemoembolization for the treatment of hepatocellular carcinoma: a multivariate analysis of prognostic factor. Hepatology. 1994;19:1115–23.
17. Bernard B, Cadranel J-F, Valla D, Escolano S, Jarlier V, Opolon P. Prognostic significance of bacterial infection in bleeding cirrhotic patients: A prospective study. Gastroenterology. 1995;108:1828–34.
18. Smith RB, Warren WD, Salam AA *et al.* Dacron interposition shunts for portal hypertension. Ann Surg. 1980;192:9–17.
19. Christensen E, Schlichting P, Fauerholdt L *et al.* Prognostic value of Child–Turcotte criteria in medically treated cirrhosis. Hepatology. 1984;4:430–5.
20. Schlichting P, Christensen E, Andersen PK *et al.* Prognostic factors in cirrhosis identified by Cox's regression model. Hepatology. 1983;3:889–95.
21. Infante-Rivard C, Esnaola S, Villeneuve JP. Clinical and statistical validity of conventional prognostic factors in predicting short-term survival among cirrhotics. Hepatology. 1987;7:660–4.
22. Albers I, Hartmann H, Bircher J, Creutzfeldt W. Superiority of the Child–Pugh classification to quantitative liver function tests for assessing prognosis of liver cirrhosis. Scand J Gastroenterol. 1989;24:269–76.

10
Portal hypertension and survival

J. BOSCH, A. ESCORSELL and J.-C. GARCÍA-PAGÁN

INTRODUCTION

Portal hypertension is a major determinant of the clinical outcome of patients with chronic liver diseases, since it is responsible for the appearance of some of the more frequent and severe complications that can develop in these patients, such as massive bleeding from ruptured gastroesophageal varices and portal hypertensive gastropathy (PHG), ascites, renal dysfunction and spontaneous bacterial peritonitis. These complications carry a poor prognosis and are leading causes of death and of liver transplantation in these patients[1].

In patients with cirrhosis, the primary factor leading to an increase in portal pressure is an increased intrahepatic vascular resistance to portal blood flow. The increased hepatic vascular resistance is primarily due to the marked distortion of the liver microvascular architecture inherent to cirrhosis, and is aggravated by an increased hepatic vascular tone, due to the active contraction of myofibroblasts and activated perisinusoidal cells. A concomitant increase in portal venous inflow and in circulating blood volume, as part of a hyperkinetic circulatory syndrome, contributes to maintain and aggravate the portal hypertension despite the formation of extensive portal–systemic collaterals, that may divert a large fraction of the portal blood flow to the systemic circulation, bypassing the liver[1,2].

Therefore, the pathophysiological events that lead to portal hypertension closely reflect the structural and functional abnormalities caused by cirrhosis and liver failure. Because of that it is conceivable that both the clinical events related to portal hypertension, as well as quantitative measurements related to the basic mechanisms involved in its pathogenesis, may be of prognostic significance in patients with chronic liver disease, and may thus be used as surrogate markers of prognosis in clinical trials.

CLINICAL MANIFESTATIONS AND NATURAL HISTORY RELATED TO PROGNOSIS

At the time of diagnosis of cirrhosis, 50% of the patients already have manifestations of portal hypertension, the more frequent being the presence of oesophageal varices. An increased portal pressure is also present in most of the remainder without any clinical consequence; these patients have a *subclinical portal hypertension.*

Several studies have assessed the rate of development of the complications of portal hypertension. Thus, the rate of formation of varices is approximately 7–8% per year (with up to 90% of patients developing varices on long-term follow-up)[3,4]; the risk of first bleeding from the varices is 20–40% at 2 years[5]; the risk of rebleeding in patients surviving the first episode of bleeding is 70% at 1 year (25–30% at 1 week)[6]; severe PHG develops in 30% of patients[7]; the risk

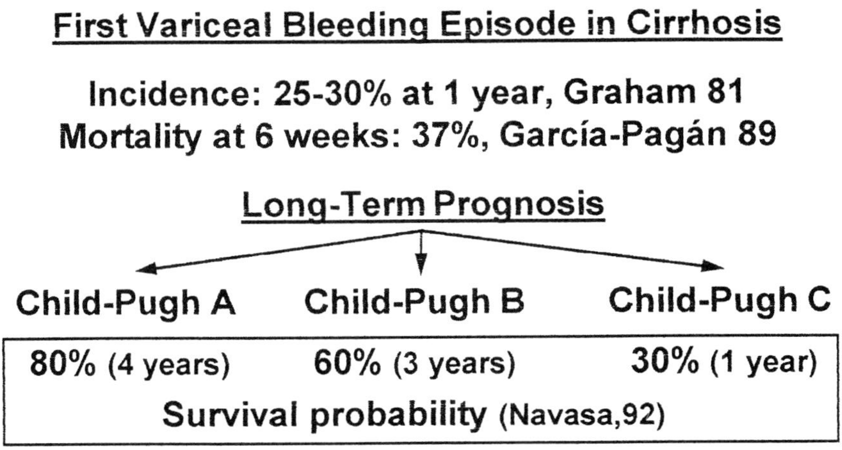

Fig. 1 Incidence and prognosis of variceal haemorrhage in patients with cirrhosis

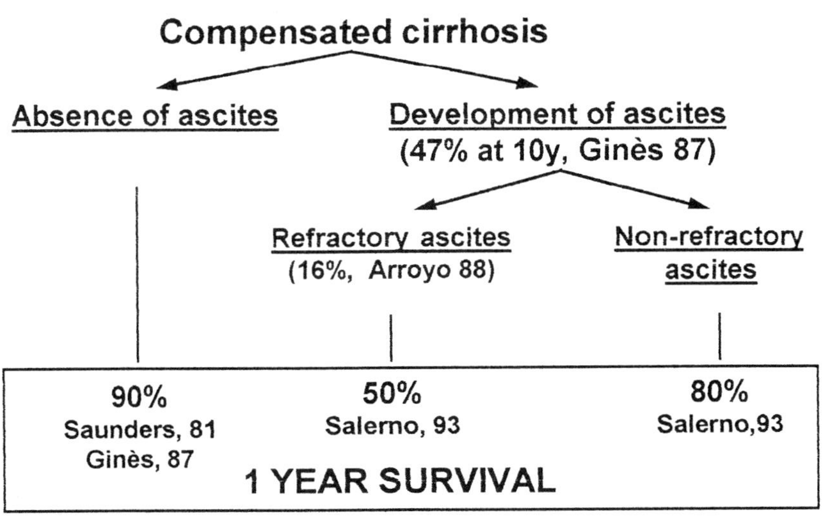

Fig. 2 Incidence and prognosis of ascites in patients with cirrhosis

- **Spontaneous bacterial peritonitis (Llach, 92)**
  - **Incidence** **11% at 1 year**
    15% at 3 years
  - **Survival** **38% at 1 year**
- **Functional renal failure (Ginès, 93)**
  - **Incidence** **18% at 1 year**
    39% at 5 years
  - **Survival** **0% at 1 year (50% at 2 weeks)**

Fig. 3 Incidence and prognosis of the complications of ascites

of developing ascites is 40% at 5 years[8]; renal dysfunction appears in 30% of these patients[9,10]; spontaneous bacterial peritonitis (SBP) appears in 15% of patients with ascites[11] and recurrence of SBP is about 70% at 1 year[12]. Each of these clinical complications of portal hypertension has a prognostic implication in terms of short and long-term survival (Figures 1–3). In many of them, the prognostic implication is very severe, including the 30% 6-week mortality of patients bleeding from varices[13] and the 50% 6-month mortality of patients with refractory ascites[14]. Therefore, there is a rational basis for the use of the complications of portal hypertension as surrogate markers of survival in patients with cirrhosis.

A very important concept that has been strongly substantiated in recent years is that the major determinant for portal hypertension to become clinically significant is that the *portal pressure gradient* (the difference between portal pressure and the free hepatic venous pressure) increases above a critical threshold value. The portal pressure gradient is most frequently assessed by measuring the hepatic venous pressure gradient (HVPG) at hepatic vein catheterization[15]. Abnormal values of the HVPG are up to 5 mm Hg. The *threshold value* of HVPG for the formation of varices is ≈10 mm Hg, and of 12 mm Hg for the appearance of clinical complications such as variceal bleeding, ascites and PHG[16–19]. Patients with an HVPG above these threshold values but without clinical complications are at high risk of developing these manifestations. HVPG has been shown to correlate with prognosis in several studies[19–21]. Therefore, the measurement of HVPG provides useful information on the natural history of portal hypertension and has potential for being used as a surrogate marker of survival.

The final, and more important determinant of survival in patients with cirrhosis and portal hypertension is the degree of liver failure[22]. This influences survival not only directly (i.e. the death rate from liver failure) but also from the complications of portal hypertension, since these are more frequent and severe in patients with advanced hepatic failure than in those with moderate impairment of liver function[23]. The degree of liver failure is usually evaluated by composite indexes – such as the Child–Pugh classification[22] and score – or by 'liver function' tests, some of which have been shown to be of prognostic significance[24,25]. Thus, both clinical data and laboratory tests may have potential as surrogate markers of prognosis in clinical trials.

DO WE NEED SURROGATE MARKERS?

The best way of assessing prognosis is to have survival/mortality as the main endpoint when designing a randomized controlled trial. However, this is very rarely done because the sample size required to assess survival is much larger (and the duration of follow-up longer) than that required to assess the impact of treatment on clinical complications. Nevertheless, investigators still want to have an idea of what could be the effect of therapy on survival, which can only be obtained by indirect methods, such as meta-analysis and/or the use of surrogate markers. Therefore, the need for use of surrogate markers arises from the failure to perform adequately designed studies.

PROS AND CONS OF SURROGATE MARKERS

Ideally, a surrogate marker should be as good at assessing prognosis as looking at the endpoint it is aimed to reflect. In practice, this is rarely the case, if ever. The usual practice is to accept as surrogate marker any parameter that has been shown to be significantly correlated with the final outcome from a statistical point of view.

However, there is always some degree of uncertainty in using these surrogate markers (Table 1). This uncertainty is the main argument against its use, and is due to several factors. The more important are:

- Inappropriate 'source studies', either because of a small sample size or because of retrospective design.
- Poor definition of the parameter used as surrogate marker. This is specially important with qualitative rather than quantitative parameters (i.e. 'presence of ascites': tense ascites requiring admission vs. ascites shown by ultrasonography).
- Use of inadequate method to assess the parameter. Very common in 'old' studies (i.e. studies where the presence of oesophageal varices was assessed radiologically).
- Use of surrogate markers in situations different from those in which they have been shown to correlate with prognosis.

Because of these many caveats, the use of surrogate markers should not be encouraged. The best use of surrogate markers is not as a substitute for direct assessment of prognosis, but as ancillary secondary endpoints, which can be very helpful in better characterizing the effects of therapy, especially when this is of borderline significance. In addition, there are specific situations where surrogate markers can be very helpful; a good example could be the development of SBP or functional renal failure in patients with ascites.

Table 1 Markers of prognosis in patients with chronic liver diseases

Class	*Marker*
First	Survival
Second	Need for liver transplantation Development of major complications related to portal hypertension: Varices and variceal bleeding Ascites Renal dysfunction Spontaneous bacterial peritonitis Hepatic encephalopathy
Third	Measurements of portal pressure gradient or HVPG Child–Pugh score
Others	Liver function tests: ABT, GEC, HCI Indirect liver decompensation tests: plasma catecholamines Specific situations: *Variceal bleeding*: transfusion requirements, endoscopic findings *Ascites*: renal failure, SBP, high PRA, low arterial pressure, low ascites protein

SPECIFIC MARKERS

Implicit in the above considerations is that not all surrogate markers of prognosis are of similar value; while some are close to what we can consider as 'first class' or 'premium markers', others can only be considered as 'third class' markers (although their value may be higher in specific situations). A short discussion of the pros and cons of these markers follows.

Survival

This is the gold standard. However, it is difficult to reach. Nevertheless, we have to insist on the importance of designing and conducting large-sized trials with enough power to assess the impact on prognosis of new treatments in patients with chronic liver disease.

Need for liver transplantation

If liver transplantation could be offered to all patients with advanced liver failure, the requirement for liver transplantation and its immediate outcome could be used as an alternative to survival in assessing prognosis. At present this is still not the case, but many authors recommend use of a combined endpoint (death or liver transplantation) to assess the impact of treatment on prognosis. Besides, because of its socio-economic relevance, the requirement for liver transplantation may be considered a main endpoint in randomized controlled trials: a treatment that can decrease the need for liver transplantation would be clinically relevant *per se* (although it will also probably result in an improvement in prognosis).

Development of complications related to portal hypertension

As already discussed, the development of the major complications of portal hypertension (such as the appearance of varices, gastrointestinal bleeding, ascites, renal dysfunction, SBP and hepatic encephalopathy) carries clear prognostic implications, which provides the basis for using these events as markers of prognosis in long-term follow-up studies. However, there is a need for clear definitions of each of these endpoints and a standardization of the methods used to verify their presence. There have been recent attempts to do so in international conferences, such as the Baveno II Meeting, and the International Ascites Club criteria for the diagnosis of refractory ascites and hepatorenal syndrome.

These complications are at the present time the major endpoints in many RCTs aimed at preventing the complications of cirrhosis[5]. These studies are obviously very interesting and potentially of great clinical relevance. However, it is still absolutely necessary to prove the impact of these treatments on prognosis. We cannot assume that if we can prevent variceal bleeding or ascites we will have a better survival. Certainly, by doing so we would prevent deaths due to bleeding or ascites, but it is possible that the overall prognosis is not improved because, for instance, of an increased death rate from liver failure or from non-liver related problems. This was the case in the early studies with prophylactic portacaval shunts. It is very important to remember that, because of the advent of new technologies, such as TIPS, portacaval shunts are again *à la mode*.

Measurement of portal pressure gradient or HVPG

There has been an increasing interest in the use of measurements of portal pressure as a marker of prognosis. This is a well defined parameter, with standardized methods of measurement[15], which has been shown to correlate with prognosis by different independent centres from different countries. Its use is encouraged, since this will provide additional information on the potential advantages of using a real 'liver test' as an indirect marker of the prognosis of chronic liver diseases[19–21]. It is possible that if this measurement had previously been available, it would have proved as useful as indirect, non-liver related prognostic markers, such as plasma renin activity or sodium excretion[11]. Interestingly, multivariate analysis has shown the hepatic vein pressure gradient (HVPG) to be as good as the Child–Pugh score as a prognostic indicator of survival[20].

On the other hand, *repeated* measurements of portal pressure gradient or of HVPG have been shown to be very valuable and accurate markers of the long-term efficacy of the treatment of portal hypertension. Specifically, Groszmann *et al.*[26] have proved that reduction of HVPG below the 12 mm Hg threshold value by pharmacological treatment is associated with total protection from the risk of variceal bleeding[26], and that even if this target is not reached, a decrease in HVPG greater than 20% of baseline values after 3 months of drug therapy is associated with an extremely low risk of rebleeding during long-term follow-up[27]. This has raised the possibility of using the HVPG response as a guide for therapeutic decisions in the treatment of portal hypertension. However, the correlation between these responses and survival has not yet been firmly established.

Child–Pugh score

The Child–Pugh score (Table 2) is a composite index for evaluation of the degree of liver failure in patients with cirrhosis. It includes clinical information (presence and degree of ascites and of hepatic encephalopathy) and quantitative biochemical data (serum bilirubin, plasma albumin and prothrombin activity). Although originally designed to assess the operative risk of portacaval shunt surgery, it has been found to be extremely useful as a marker of prognosis in many different situations. Despite being largely empirical, this is the best prognostic indicator in patients with cirrhosis (better than 'quantitative' liver function tests). Its accuracy improves by using the numerical score rather than the A,B,C groups.

In longitudinal studies, it is likely that changes in the Child–Pugh score can be used as surrogate markers of long-term prognosis. Besides, its well-known prognostic value ensures that control and interventional groups in RCTs in patients with cirrhosis are well matched with regard to the Child–Pugh score. Many RCTs actually choose to stratify the patients according to this parameter.

Miscellaneous

Liver function tests

Some of the so-called 'liver function tests' exhibit a good correlation with survival, and therefore may be used as surrogate markers or in assessing comparability of

Table 2 Clinical assessment of the degree of liver failure (Child–Pugh score)[a]

Parameter	*Range*	*Points*
Encephalopathy (grade)	Absent	1
	I and II	2
	III and IV	3
Ascites	Absent	1
	Mild	2
	Tense	3
Bilirubin (mg/dl)[b]	<2	1
	2–3	2
	>3	3
Albumin (g/dl)	>3.5	1
	2.8–3.5	2
	<2.8	3
Prothrombin ratio (%)	>50	1
	30–50	2
	<30	3
	Group A: 5–6 points Group B: 7–9 points Group C: 10–15 points	

[a]The original Child's classification included nutritional status evaluated as excellent, fair and poor instead of prothrombin ratio

[b]Correction for bilirubin in primary biliary cirrhosis: <4 mg/dl (1 point); 4–10 mg/dl (2 points); >10 mg/dl (3 points)

(From reference 22)

different treatment groups. The best is the serum bilirubin level, which is the strongest biochemical parameter included in the Child–Pugh score. Serum bilirubin is also extremely useful for assessment of prognosis in primary biliary cirrhosis.

More interesting is the use of 'quantitative' or 'semi-quantitative' liver function tests, which have been specifically developed in the hope that they would be as successful as nephrological parameters such as GFR and serum creatinine. The more popular tests have been the galactose-elimination capacity (GEC)[28], the aminopyrine breath test (ABT)[29] and the hepatic clearance of ICG (ICG-Cl)[24,25,30]. All these tests have been shown to correlate with prognosis in different studies, although they are all expensive, cumbersome and have no clear advantages over the Child–Pugh score in most situations. However, serial measurements of the GEC have been shown to allow a very good estimation of prognosis in PBC, and the ICG-Cl has been shown to be better than the Child–Pugh score in assessing the prognosis in patients that have survived variceal haemorrhage[25]. The MEGX test has been the most recent introduction[31]. It would be desirable for large RCTs to include some of these tests to verify whether repeated measurements allow a reasonable prediction of death; this would permit use these tests as surrogate markers of prognosis.

Indirect parameters reflecting the severity of liver decompensation

Several studies have shown that some parameters, not directly related to liver disease, have prognostic value in patients with cirrhosis. Most of them reflect the severity of liver decompensation, such as arterial hypotension and increased plasma noradrenaline and adrenaline concentrations[21]. These parameters should be used with caution in prognosis, since they can be affected by the treatment modality or by the conditions of measurement.

Specific situations

Some specific situations may use specific surrogate markers. In variceal bleeding episodes, for example, parameters such as transfusion requirements, need for surgical intervention, and endoscopic findings may be of interest[13]. Similarly, in patients with ascites, several studies have shown that parameters reflecting neurohumoral abnormalities and renal impairment (renal failure, increased PRA, increased noradrenaline, low urinary sodium excretion, low arterial pressure) correlate closely with prognosis[10,14]. These parameters should be used with care: the increased urinary sodium concentration caused by diuretics does not indicate an improvement in prognosis, neither does the rise in plasma renin activity imply a poor prognosis. In patients with ascites, a low ascites protein concentration indicates an increased risk of spontaneous bacterial peritonitis[11]. Again, it should be remembered that ascites protein may change due to treatment; it increases, for example, during diuresis.

Acknowledgements

Supported by grants from the Fondo de Investigaciones Sanitarias (FIS 94/0757) and Dirección General de Investigación Científica y Tecnológica (DGICYT PB94-1562).

References

1. Bosch J, García-Pagán JC, Feu F, Rodés J. Portal hypertension: Clinical pathobiology. In: Arias IM, Boyer JL, Fausto N, Jakoby WB, Schachter D, editors. The liver. Biology and pathobiology, 3rd ed. New York: Raven Press, 1994:1343–55.
2. Bosch J, Pizcueta P, Feu F, Fernández M, García-Pagán JC. Pathophysiology of portal hypertension. Gastroenterol Clin North Am. 1992;21:1–14.
3. Pagliaro L, D'Amico G, Pasta L *et al.* Portal hypertension in cirrhosis: Natural history. In: Bosch J, Groszmann RJ, editors. Portal hypertension. Pathophysiology and treatment. Oxford: Blackwell Scientific, 1994:72–92.
4. Calès P, Desmorat H, Vinel JP *et al.* Incidence of large oesophageal varices in patients with cirrhosis: Application to prophylaxis of first bleeding. Gut. 1990;31:1298–302.
5. D'Amico G, Pagliaro L, Bosch J. The treatment of portal hypertension: A meta-analytic review. Hepatology. 1995;22:332–54.
6. Graham DY, Smith JL. The course of patients following variceal hemorrhage. Gastroenterology. 1981;80:800–9.
7. D'Amico G, Montalbano L, Traina M *et al.* Natural history of congestive gastropathy in cirrhosis. Gastroenterology. 1990;99:1558–64.
8. Ginés P, Quintero E, Arroyo V *et al.* Compensated cirrhosis: Natural history and prognostic factors. Hepatology. 1987;7:122–8.
9. Ginés A, Escorsell A, Ginès P *et al.* Incidence, predictive factors, and prognosis of the hepatorenal syndrome in cirrhosis with ascites. Gastroenterology. 1993;105:229–36.
10. Llach J, Ginès P, Arroyo V *et al.* Prognostic value of arterial pressure, endogenous vasoactive systems, and renal function in cirrhosis patients admitted to the hospital for the treatment of ascites. Gastroenterology. 1988;94:482–7.
11. Llach J, Rimola A, Navasa M *et al.* Incidence and predictive factors of first episode of spontaneous bacterial peritonitis in cirrhosis with ascites: Relevance of ascitic fluid protein concentration. Hepatology. 1992;16:724–7.
12. Titó Ll, Rimola A, Ginès P, Llach J, Arroyo V, Rodés J. Recurrence of spontaneous bacterial peritonitis in cirrhosis: Frequency and predictive factors. Hepatology. 1988;8:27–31.
13. García-Pagán JC, Terés J, Calvet X, Bosch J, Rodés J. Factors which influence the prognosis of the first episode of variceal hemorrhage in patients with cirrhosis. In: Bosch EJ, Rodés J, editors. Recent advances in the pathophysiology and therapy of portal hypertension. Serono, Symposia Review No. 22, 1989:287–302.
14. Salerno F, Borroni G, Moser P *et al.* Survival and prognostic factors of cirrhotic patients with ascites: A study of 134 outpatients. Am J Gastroenterol. 1993;88:514–9.
15. Bosch J, Mastai R, Kravetz D, Navasa M, Rodés J. Hemodynamic evaluation of the patient with portal hypertension. Sem Liver Dis. 1986;6:309–17.
16. Lebrec D, DeFleury P, Rueff B, Nahum H, Benhamou JP. Portal hypertension, size of esophageal varices and risk of gastrointestinal bleeding in alcoholic cirrhosis. Gastroenterology. 1980;79:1139–44.
17. Garcia-Tsao G, Groszmann RJ, Fisher RL, Conn HO, Atterbury CE, Glickman M. Portal pressure presence of gastroesophageal varices and variceal bleeding. Hepatology. 1985;5:419–24.
18. Viallet A, Marleau D, Huet M *et al.* Hemodynamic evaluation of patients with intrahepatic portal hypertension: Relationship between bleeding varices and the portohepatic gradient. Gastroenterology. 1975;69:1297–300.
19. García-Pagán JC, Bosch J. Clinical-hemodynamic correlates in the evaluation and treatment of portal hypertensión. In: Rodés J, Arroyo V, Bosch J. editors. Treatments in liver disease. International Meeting on Therapy in Liver Disease, Barcelona: Masson, 1995:33–40.
20. Merkel C, Bolognesi M, Bellon S *et al.* Prognostic usefulness of hepatic vein catheterization in patients with cirrhosis and esophageal varices. Gastroenterology. 1992;102:973–9.
21. Tage-Jensen U, Henriksen JH, Christensen E, Widding A, Ring-Larsen H, Christensen NJ. Plasma catecholamine level and portal venous pressure as guides to prognosis in patients with cirrhosis. J Hepatol. 1988;6:350–8.
22. Pugh RNH, Murray-Lyon IM, Dawson JL, Pietroni MC, Williams R. Transection of the esophagus for bleeding esophageal varices. Br J Surg. 1973;60:646–9.

23. The North Italian Endoscopic Club for the study and treatment of esophageal varices. Prediction of the first variceal hemorrhage in patients with cirrhosis of the liver and esophageal varices. N Engl J Med. 1988;319:983–9.
24. Merkel C, Bolognesi M, Finucci GF *et al.* Indocyanine green intrinsic hepatic clearance as a prognostic index of survival in patients with cirrhosis. J Hepatol. 1989;9:16–22.
25. Navasa M, García-Pagán JC, Bosch J, Rodés J. Valor pronóstico del aclaramiento hepático del verde de indocianina en pacientes con cirrosis hepática y hemorragia por varices esofágicas. Med Clin (Barc). 1992;98:290–4.
26. Groszmann RJ, Bosch J, Grace ND *et al.* Hemodynamic events in a prospective randomized trial of propanolol vs placebo in the prevention of a first variceal hemorrhage. Gastroenterology. 1990;99:1401–7.
27. Feu F, García-Pagán JC, Luca A, Terés J, Bosch J, Rodés J. Clinical hemodynamic correlations during pharmacological prevention of variceal rebleeding in cirrhosis. Lancet. 1995;346:1056–9.
28. Keiding S. Galactose clearance measurements and liver blood flow. Gastroenterology. 1988;94:477–81.
29. Villeneuve JP, Infante Rivard C, Ampelas M *et al.* Prognostic value of the aminopyrine breath test in cirrhotic patients. Hepatology. 1986;6:928–31.
30. Caesar J, Shaldon S, Chiandussi L, Guevara L, Sherlock S. The use of indocyanine green in the measurement of hepatic blood flow and as a test of hepatic function. Clin Sci. 1961;21:43–57.
31. Oellerich M, Raude E, Burdelski M *et al.* Monoethylglycycinexylidide formation kinetics: A novel approach to assessment of liver function. J Clin Chem Clin Biochem. 1987;25:845–53.

11
Impact of ascites on survival of patients with liver cirrhosis

M. BERNARDI, P. CARACENI, F. TREVISANI, G. SICA, A. COLANTONI and A. GASBARRINI

INTRODUCTION

Ascites is the most frequent complication of compensated liver cirrhosis[1] with an incidence ranging from 5 to 10% per year[1,2]. In our experience[3], ascites is the main cause (42%) of hospitalization of patients with cirrhosis and very often contributes to the prolongation of the hospital stay. Therefore, it represents a major clinical problem.

The appearance of ascites represents a landmark in the natural history of cirrhosis and holds a precise prognostic meaning. According to different studies, the 5-year survival of cirrhotic patients without ascites varies from 45 to 80%, while it drops to 15–40% in the presence of ascites[1,2,4–7] (Figure 1). Moreover, ascites has often been found to be an independent risk factor for mortality[8]. Finally, the presence of ascites often leads to a deterioration of the working and relational life, need of repeated hospital admissions as in- and out-patients, and chronic treatments.

FACTORS RELATED TO POOR PROGNOSIS OF ASCITES

There are many reasons for the adverse prognostic meaning of cirrhotic ascites. First, ascites appears when pathogenetic factors, such as abnormalities in liver function, portal and systemic haemodynamics, and renal function, have reached a critical threshold severity[9]. Even worse, the same factors also lead to life-threatening events, including gastrointestinal bleeding, encephalopathy or renal failure. Thus, it is not surprising that these factors proved to be independent prognostic indicators for mortality in many studies[8]. Second, ascites itself induces additional complications, closely linked to its presence, such as spontaneous bacterial peritonitis, restrictive respiratory failure, or rupture of

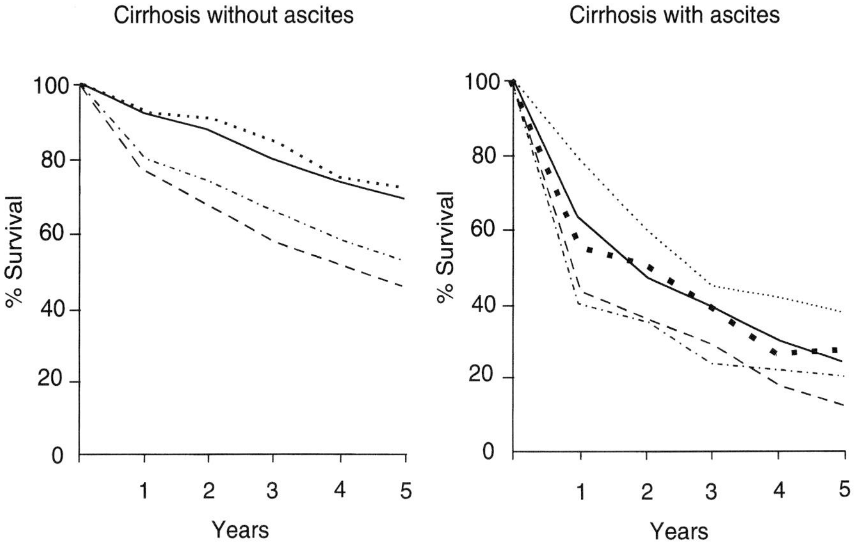

Fig. 1 Five-year survival of cirrhotic patients with and without ascites. Data are derived from different studies: Ginés *et al.* (reference 1); D'Amico *et al.* (reference 2); Saunders *et al.* (reference 4); Christensen *et al.* (reference 5); Llach *et al.* (reference 6); and Salerno *et al.* (reference 7) (modified from Pagliaro and Simonetti, reference 63)

abdominal hernias. Finally, ascites implies pharmacological or invasive treatments which can lead to further morbidity or even to death.

Pathogenetic factors

A detailed review of the pathogenesis of ascites is beyond the scope of this book. It can be recalled, however, that the development of ascites is the result of the combination of 'local' factors, such as portal hypertension and reduced colloid osmotic pressure secondary to hypoalbuminaemia, and 'systemic' factors, such as reduced effective volaemia, hyperdynamic circulation and renal retention of sodium and water[9].

It is still unclear whether the impairment of liver function by itself is a major pathogenetic factor promoting renal sodium retention and ascites[10,11]. In any case, there is no doubt that the residual liver function of cirrhotics with ascites is poorer than that of compensated patients, and many indicators of liver function, such as serum bilirubin[1,7,12,13], prothrombin time[1,2,12], serum albumin[1,7,12,13], galactose elimination capacity[14], aminopyrine breath test[14–16], indocyanine green test[14,17] and monoethyleneglycinexylidide (MEGX) test[17] have been found to be independent prognostic indicators of mortality in several studies.

A number of studies have shown that the degree of portal hypertension, as evaluated by porto-hepatic gradient[18] or wedged-to-free hepatic venous pressure gradient[19,20], is directly correlated with mortality in patients with cirrhosis. Indeed, ascites only appears once a critical value of portal hypertension has been reached, being virtually absent with a portal pressure, as evaluated by wedged hepatic vein pressure, below 15 mm Hg[21]. A similar threshold is also associated with bleeding from gastroesophageal varices and hypertensive gastropathy[22,23]. Therefore, it is not surprising that patients with ascites carry a greater risk of bleeding as compared to those without ascites[24,25]. In fact, up to one-third of the former will bleed within two years, while this complication only occurs in 15% of patients with compensated cirrhosis. Even worse, the presence of ascites brings a higher mortality in bleeding patients[25]. Such a greater mortality is probably related to the haemostatic imbalance[26], the severe circulatory abnormalities with reduced cardiovascular responsiveness[27], and the elevated operative risk[28], which mark the advanced stages of the liver disease. Moreover, gastrointestinal bleeding in patients with ascites can precipitate spontaneous bacterial peritonitis[29].

The link between ascites formation and reduced serum albumin concentration is far less clear than with the degree of portal hypertension. Nonetheless, Wood *et al.* found that serum albumin concentration below 35 g/L predicted the presence of ascites in 83% of cases[30], and a colloid osmotic pressure of 20 mm Hg has been found to be the threshold value below which ascites is invariably present[21]. Again, serum albumin level has been found to be an independent predictive factor for survival[1,7,12,13].

The main systemic event associated with ascites formation is the renal retention of sodium and water. This is ultimately caused by a reduction in effective blood volume, which, in turn, primes the activation of vasoconstrictor and sodium retaining systems (renin–angiotensin–aldosterone, sympathoadrenergic, arginine–vasopressin[31]), justifies the trend to low arterial pressure which characterizes patients with advanced cirrhosis[32], and impairs renal perfusion up to functional renal failure[33]. In recent years, many parameters influenced by cardiovascular and renal function, such as plasma renin activity[34], plasma noradrenaline concentration[6,20], mean arterial pressure[6], renal sodium excretion[6,34], creatinine clearance[6], and free water clearance[35], have been found to be independent prognostic indicators of mortality in cirrhosis. Interestingly, these factors often succeed in determining prognosis even in patients with a very advanced stage of cirrhosis, when classical parameters reflecting liver function have already lost their predictive value.

Complications directly related to the presence of ascites

Spontaneous bacterial peritonitis (SBP) only arises in patients with ascites. It is favoured by a low protein concentration in the ascitic fluid[36–38] and can be precipitated by gastrointestinal bleeding[29]. In hospitalized patients, its prevalence varies from 10 to 27%[37,39], and its one-year incidence ranges between 8 and 20%[40,41]. SBP carries a very poor prognosis, the short-term mortality still being around 17–50%[41–43]. Moreover, it recurs in about 70% of cases within one year[44]. Although antibiotic prophylaxis using different regimens succeeds in preventing the occurrence or recurrence of SBP, the long-term survival of patients is not significantly improved[45,46]. Thus, SBP still represents an ominous complication, which negatively and strongly affects the survival of patients with ascites, despite the substantial progresses in diagnosis, treatment and prophylaxis made in recent years.

The incidence of other complications closely linked with the presence of massive ascites, such as reduced ventilation and strangulation or rupture of abdominal hernias, is not clearly defined. Nonetheless, both events can have severe consequences, given the arterial oxygen desaturation due to hepatopulmonary syndrome[47] and the very high risk of emergency surgery in patients with advanced cirrhosis[28].

Complications of treatment of ascites

Up to 26% of patients with cirrhosis and ascites treated by dietary sodium restriction and diuretics can develop renal failure[48]. This condition usually resolves and, therefore, carries a relatively good prognosis in the short term provided that it is promptly recognized and corrected. Other complications which can be induced by diuretic treatment include encephalopathy, hypokalaemia and hyponatraemia[49].

When the use of diuretics becomes unfeasible, other more invasive treatments are needed to manage ascites, such as paracentesis[50], ascites reinfusion techniques[51,52], peritoneovenous shunts[53,54], and transjugular intrahepatic porto–systemic shunts (TIPSS)[55]. Although the safety of paracentesis has been established by clinical trials and current practice, it can represent a direct cause of ascitic fluid infection and intraperitoneal haemorrhage. The complications of ascites reinfusion techniques or peritoneovenous shunting can also be important, and some of them life threatening, such as disseminated intravascular coagulation, left ventricular failure, bleeding from oesophageal varices, superior vena cava thrombosis and sepsis[56,57]. The use of TIPSS for the treatment of refractory ascites still awaits worldwide acceptance, but it is more and more frequently employed in such cases. Although it would appear effective in relieving refractory ascites, several studies have shown that TIPSS insertion can be followed by the onset or worsening of encephalopathy and liver failure[58].

CIRRHOSIS WITH ASCITES: A HETEROGENEOUS POPULATION

There is no doubt that ascites represents a reliable negative prognostic factor. However, as already mentioned in the introduction, the 5-year mortality of patients with cirrhosis and ascites greatly varies, ranging from 15% to 40% in different studies. Such a variability may represent a confounding element in the interpretation of the investigations dealing with either natural history of the disease or the effects of various forms of treatment. A comment on the heterogeneity of patient populations identified as ‘carrying ascites’ is therefore warranted. In fact, this definition encompasses individuals very different from each other in terms of pathophysiological background and clinical presentation[59].

‘Spontaneous’ and ‘precipitated’ ascites

The clinical background underlying the first ascitic decompensation is relevant to determine patient prognosis. In many cases, ascites is temporarily associated with a well identifiable precipitating factor. In our experience, these events were recognized, alone or in combination, in 65% of the patients admitted with ascites: gastrointestinal bleeding (31%), infection (29%), alcohol abuse (20%), hepatic or renal drug-induced toxicity (17%), surgery (11%), excessive dietary sodium intake (11%), and extrahepatic cholestasis (6%). Although these conditions prime ascitic decompensation by acting through different mechanisms (impairment of renal and cardiovascular functions, volume overload, liver failure), they have in common the fact that they can be eliminated or resolved. If this happens, ascites can disappear, and a certain number of these patients eventually enter even a prolonged period of 'compensation.'

In other instances, ascites develops in the absence of a clearly identifiable precipitating event. In these cases, decompensation probably occurs because a critical threshold is reached by the interplay of the pathogenetic factors. In other words, this event marks a 'point-of-no-return' in the evolution of the disease, beyond which ascites can only be controlled by means of chronic therapy.

It remains to be established whether such clinically and pathogenetically different presentations of ascites also imply a different prognosis. We have retrospectively evaluated the clinical records of 150 patients with ascites consecutively admitted to our institution. In 52 cases no precipitating event was identifiable (spontaneous ascites; group 1), while there was a precipitating event

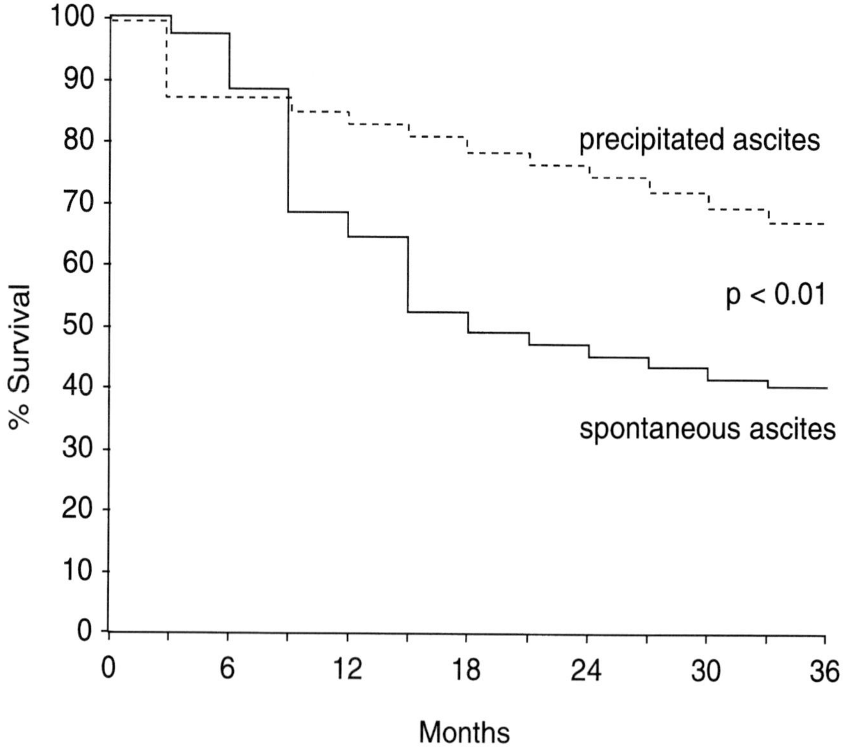

Fig. 2 Retrospective evaluation of three-year survival of patients with cirrhosis and 'precipitated' (98 patients) or 'spontaneous' (52 patients) ascites

in the remainder (group 2). The mortality during the first hospital stay was 4% in group 1 and 13% in group 2, while the 3-year mortality was 41% and 66%, respectively (Figure 2). Based on these observations, it appears that 'spontaneous' and 'precipitated' ascites are far from being a homogeneous entity, and their grouping in prognostic studies or therapeutic trials may be misleading. It would be advisable for patients with 'precipitated' ascites only to be included in such studies once it has been established that ascitic decompensation persists even after the resolution of the precipitating event.

Firstly developed and long-standing ascites

The pathogenetic background underlying the first ascitic decompensation and a long-standing ascites, regardless of the responsiveness to diuretic therapy, is often quite different. In fact, when ascites first appears, renal perfusion is usually preserved, and the activation of vasoconstrictor and sodium-retaining systems, such as the renin–aldosterone axis and the sympathetic nervous system, is mild or even absent. In contrast, patients with long-standing ascites usually show impaired renal perfusion and a marked hyperactivity of neurohumoral factors promoting renal sodium retention and attempting to counterbalance arterial vasodilation[33,60,61] (Figure 3). In addition, liver function impairment is generally

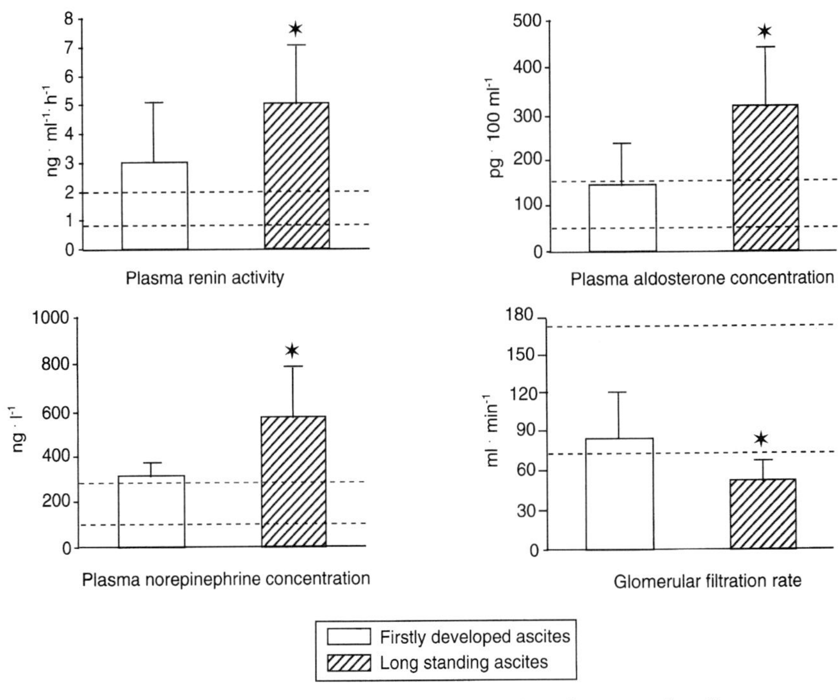

Fig. 3 Plasma renin activity, plasma aldosterone concentration, plasma noradrenaline concentration and glomerular filtration rate in patients with firstly developed ascites (empty bars, 21 patients) and long-standing ascites (hatched bars, 25 patients). *: $p<0.05$ or lower

more severe than in patients who present ascites for the first time. We have already mentioned that renal function, plasma renin activity, plasma noradrenaline concentration and other factors, directly or indirectly related with ascites formation, have been proved to be independent prognostic factors in patients with ascites. Thus, the survival of patients with long-standing and first-appeared ascites could be quite different, and their relative proportion in a patient population may affect the results of an investigation and, in particular, the survival rate. Therefore, a correct patient enrolment should take into account these two main entities when a study on ascitic patients is planned. In any case, to report the relative proportion of long-standing and first-appeared ascites would allow the reader proper data interpretation.

Tense and refractory ascites

Many clinical trials have been performed on patients with 'tense ascites'. This term typically identifies a patient population with massive peritoneal effusion. Sometimes, tense (or massive) ascites is also used or felt as synonymous with

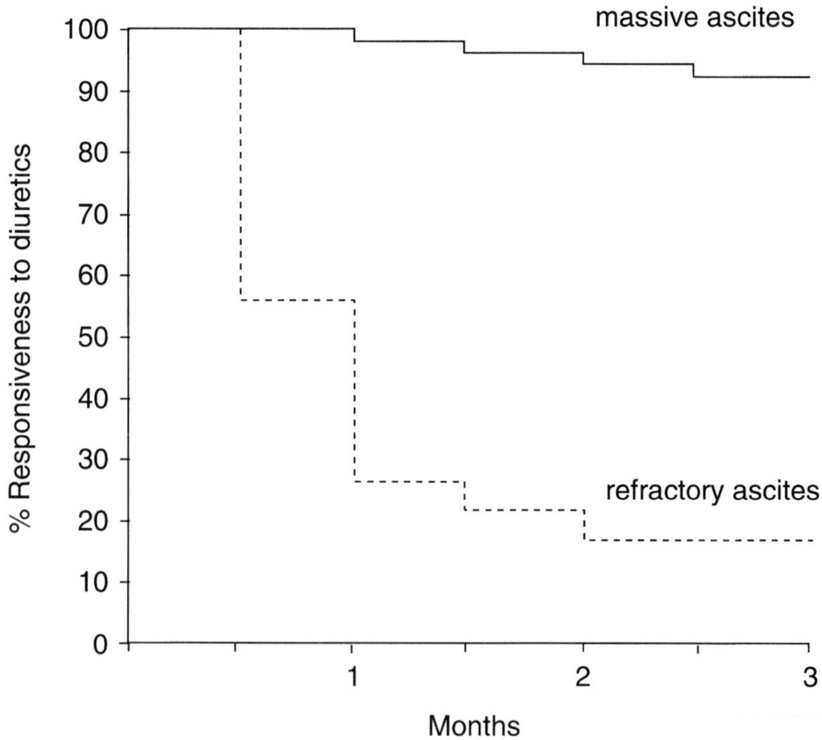

Fig. 4 Responsiveness to diuretic treatment in patients with tense ascites during a three-month follow-up after ascites removal by paracentesis or ascites apheresis, concentration and reinfusion. Patients fulfilling the criteria for refractory ascites according to Arroyo *et al.* (reference 62) were classified as 'refractory ascites' (16 patients), the remainder as 'massive ascites' (24 patients)

refractory ascites. However, only some of these patients really present with refractory ascites, while, in the remainder, even a massive ascites can ultimately be treated with medical therapy. In our experience, by applying the definition of refractory ascites proposed by an international working team[62], no more than 40% of massive ascites were also refractory. Further evidence that these conditions differ both pathophysiologically and clinically is provided by the observation that after ascites removal by paracentesis or using the technique of apheresis, concentration and reinfusion of the ascitic fluid[52], more than 90% of patients with massive ascites were successfully managed with diuretics for at least 3 months, while this only happened in 14% of patients with refractory ascites (Figure 4). The correct definition of refractory ascites is not only important for the correct interpretation of the results of therapeutic trials, but is also relevant in terms of prognosis. In fact, the survival of patients with refractory ascites is significantly shorter than that of patients with treatable ascites[7,63] (Figure 5).

Ascites and hepatorenal syndrome

The cumulative probability of developing hepatorenal syndrome (HRS) in patients with cirrhosis and ascites is 18% at one year and 39% at 5 years[64]. This complication refers to a functional renal failure, which, in contrast with classical

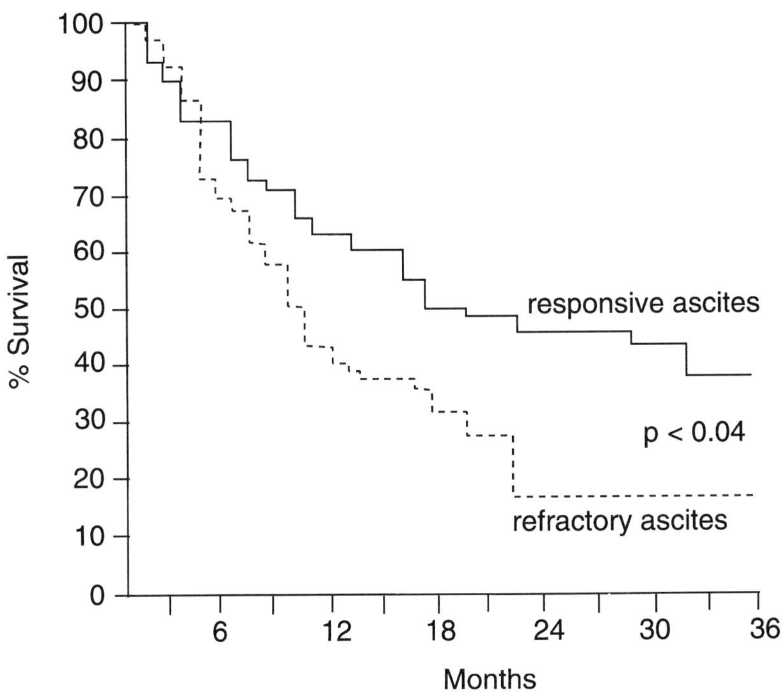

Fig. 5 Three-year survival of patients with cirrhosis and ascites responsive (51 patients) or refractory (56 patients) to diuretic therapy (modified from Pagliaro and Simonetti, reference 63)

pre-renal uraemia, is not resolved by plasma volume expansion. It is characterized by an intense vasoconstriction of the renal arteries, leading to the reduction of renal blood flow and glomerular filtration rate in the absence of identifiable causes of renal failure[65]. Virtually all patients with HRS present refractory ascites. HRS can be seen as the extreme consequence of the circulatory imbalance of cirrhosis[9] and, therefore, is associated with arterial hypotension and maximal activation of vasoconstrictor systems. In a recent study[65], plasma renin activity and hyponatraemia, besides the absence of hepatomegaly, were found to be independent predictive factors for the development of the syndrome. No wonder, therefore, that prognosis of patients with HRS is extremely poor: almost 90% of patients die within 10 weeks of diagnosis, the median survival being as short as 1.7 weeks[65].

IMPACT OF ASCITES ON THE OUTCOME OF ORTHOTOPIC LIVER TRANSPLANTATION

Due to its adverse prognostic meaning, patients with cirrhosis and ascites should be considered for orthotopic liver transplantation. In this context, ascites maintains an important prognostic value, since it appears to be linked with early postoperative renal impairment and mortality[66,67]. In one study, ascites was identified as one of the seven variables associated with a significantly increased risk for death[66]. In another cohort of patients surviving beyond 72 hours after liver transplantation, 72% of those who died during the subsequent follow-up had preoperative ascites, which, in contrast, was present in 52% of survivors[67]. Although this difference was not statistically significant, preoperative ascites was among the variables predicting the occurrence of early postoperative renal impairment, which was present in all but one of the 25 patients who died. Finally, preoperative ascites and renal sodium retention are associated with major blood loss during orthotopic liver transplantation[68].

IMPACT OF THE TREATMENT OF ASCITES ON SURVIVAL

Although the presence of ascites is beyond any doubt an important negative prognostic factor for mortality of patients with cirrhosis, survival does not appear to be influenced by the different treatments. Over the last few years, several randomized controlled studies performed in large series of patients have evaluated the impact of the use of diuretics, paracentesis and peritoneovenous shunt on survival.

In the first controlled trial comparing the effects of paracentesis plus i.v. albumin and diuretic treatment, Ginés *et al.*[50] showed that, despite the former being more effective in removing ascites, the 2-year survival of patients did not significantly differ, being approximately 40 vs. 45%. Similar figures can be found in other studies, which evaluated the effects of paracentesis associated with the infusion of albumin or artificial plasma expanders[69–71]. When medical therapy and peritoneovenous shunting were compared, 2-year survival rates were about 60% for patients with ‘normal or mild abnormalities of liver function tests' and 33% for those with 'more severe liver dysfunction or previous complications', regardless of the kind of treatment[53]. Similarly, the 3-year survival rate was 34% in patients treated with paracentesis associated with albumin infusion as compared to 33% for patients undergoing peritoneovenous shunting[54]. Even a technical improvement of the LeVeen shunt by using titanium tip at the jugular end to prevent caval thrombosis, did not change such figures[72]. Whether the placement of TIPSS would succeed in improving the survival of patients with refractory ascites has yet to be established.

It is clear, therefore, that different treatments do not affect the survival of patients with ascites. Even worse, the long-term survival rates reported by the above cited investigations do not appear substantially improved with respect to those which emerge from the studies performed over the last half-century[73]. This finding clearly indicates that the successful treatment of ascites does not mean the cure of the underlying disease, which remains the real determinant of the fate of patients.

Nonetheless, careful treatment of ascites bears important clinical implications by improving the quality of life, reducing the number and the length of hospitalizations, and preventing complications directly related to the presence of the peritoneal effusion. In a recently published series where shunt surgery for variceal bleeding was compared to sclerotherapy or staple transection, the incidence of ascites, SBP and HRS, along with the number of readmissions and the total time spent in hospital were greatly reduced after surgery[74]. Although shunting did not improve survival, it had a positive impact on the natural history of ascites and, presumably, on the quality of life of the patients and costs for their management.

CONCLUSION

Ascites represents an easily identifiable sign which conveys important clinical messages. Ascites is often the direct cause of hospitalization, prolongs the hospital stay, and, by itself, can lead to significant morbidity. The problems related to its management frequently dominate the clinical setting. Even more important, ascites clearly marks the evolution of cirrhosis and the patient prognosis for survival definitely changes after its appearance. Moreover, pre-operative ascites is associated with poorer outcome of liver transplantation. Such an important meaning derives from the fact that ascites formation is linked with a number of pathogenetic events which encompass the deterioration of residual liver function, the development of severe post-sinusoidal portal hypertension, the occurrence of derangements in fluid and cardiovascular homeostasis, and the impairment of renal function. In this respect, ascites may be seen as a great surrogate marker of a series of events closely related to the progression of cirrhosis, many of which cannot be promptly and accurately assessed in current clinical practice. Based on these considerations, the presence of ascites and its evolution has to be carefully weighed up in every study aimed to define survival of patients with cirrhosis and the effects of different treatments. However, categorizing patients as 'bearing ascites' does not allow us to identify a homogeneous population with a clear cut prognosis. Nevertheless, clinical assessment and simple laboratory investigations can help us to reach a more precise characterization of these patients. Precipitated versus spontaneously appearing ascites, firstly appeared versus long-standing ascites, massive or tense versus truly refractory ascites, and ascites with preserved versus impaired renal perfusion, delineate different categories which should be considered when planning survival studies and clinical trials. In any case, the reader shall pay careful attention to such categories in order to interpret the results of these studies correctly and evaluate their applicability to clinical practice.

References

1. Ginés P, Quintero E, Arroyo V *et al.* Compensated cirrhosis: Natural history and prognostic factors. Hepatology. 1987;7:122–8.
2. D'Amico G, Morabito A, Pagliaro L *et al.* Survival and prognostic indicators in compensated and decompensated cirrhosis. Dig Dis Sci. 1986;31:468–75.
3. Bernardi M. Trattamento dell'ascite nel paziente con cirrosi epatica. BIMS. 1995;56:30–42.
4. Saunders JB, Walters JRF, Davies P, Paton A. A 20-year prospective study of cirrhosis. Br Med J. 1981;282:263–6.
5. Christensen E, Schlichhting P, Fauerholdt L *et al.* Prognostic value of Child–Turcotte criteria in medically treated cirrhosis. Hepatology. 1984;4:430–5.
6. Llach J, Ginés P, Arroyo V *et al.* Prognostic value of arterial pressure, endogenous vasoactive systems and renal function in cirrhotic patients admitted to the hospital for the treatment of ascites. Gastroenterology. 1988;94:482–7.
7. Salerno F, Borroni G, Moser P *et al.* Survival and prognostic factors of cirrhotic patients with ascites: A study of 134 outpatients. Am J Gastroenterol. 1993;88:514–9.
8. Pagliaro L, Pasta L, D'Amico G, Pulco A, Politi F, Vizzini G. Natural history of cirrhosis: Predictors of death risk, overview of published studies and validation in a new test set. In: Dobrilla G, Felder M, De Pretis F, editors. Advances in hepatobiliary and pancreatic disease. Lancaster, UK: Kluwer Academic, 1995:82–93.
9. Bernardi M, Trevisani F, Colantoni A, Gasbarrini A, De Notariis S, Gasbarrini G. Pathophysiology of ascites and hepatorenal syndrome. In: Holstege A, Schölmerich J, Hahn EG, editors. Portal hypertension. Lancaster, UK: Kluwer Academic, 1995:193–208.
10. Wensing G, Sabra R, Branch RA. The onset of sodium retention in experimental cirrhosis in rats is related to a critical threshold of liver function. Hepatology. 1990;11:779–86.
11. Rector WG Jr, Lewis F, Robertson A, Everson GT. Renal sodium retention complicating alcoholic liver disease: Relation to portosystemic shunting and liver function. Hepatology. 1990;12:455–9.
12. Christensen E, Schlichting P, Andersen PK *et al.* Updating prognosis and therapeutic effect evaluation in cirrhosis with Cox's multiple regression model for time-dependent variables. Scand J Gastroenterol. 1986;21:163–74.
13. Realdi G, Fattovich G, Hadziyannis S *et al.* Survival and prognostic factors in 366 patients with compensated cirrhosis type B: A multicenter study. J Hepatol. 1994;21:656–66.
14. Merkel C, Gatta A, Zoli M *et al.* Prognostic value of galactose elimination capacity, aminopyrine breath test and ICG clearance in patients with cirrhosis. Comparison with the Pugh Score. Dig Dis Sci. 1991;36:1197–203.
15. Merkel C, Bolognesi M, Bellon S *et al.* Aminopyrine breath test in the prognostic evaluation of patients with cirrhosis. Gut. 1992;33:836–42.
16. Villeneuve JP, Infante-Rivard C, Ampelas M, Pomier-Layrargues G, Huet PM, Maricau D. Prognostic value of aminopyrin breath test in cirrhotic patients. Hepatology. 1986;6:928–31.
17. Oellerich M, Burdelski M, Lautz HU, Binder L, Pichlmayr R. Predictors of one year pretransplant survival in patients with cirrhosis. Hepatology. 1991;14:1029–34.
18. Vinel JP, Cassigneul J, Louis A, Levade M, Pascal JP. Clinical and prognostic significance of portohepatic gradient in patients with cirrhosis. Surg Gynecol Obst. 1982;155:347–52.
19. Gluud C, Henriksen JH, Nielsen G *et al.* Prognostic indicators in alcoholic cirrhotic men. Hepatology. 1988;8:222–7.
20. Tage-Jensen U, Henriksen JH, Christensen E *et al.* Plasma catecholamine level and portal venous pressure as guides to prognosis in patients with cirrhosis. J Hepatol. 1988;6:350–8.

21. Henriksen JH, Stage GJ, Schlichting P, Winkler K. Intraperitoneal pressure: Ascitic fluid and splanchnic vascular pressures, and their role in prevention and formation of ascites. Scand J Clin Lab Invest. 1980;40:493–502.
22. Garcia-Tsao G, Grozsmann RJ, Fisher RL, Conn HO, Atterbury CE, Glickman M. Portal pressure and gastroesophageal varices bleeding. Hepatology. 1985;5:419–24.
23. Rigau J, Bosch J, Bordas JM *et al.* Endoscopic measurement of variceal pressure in cirrhosis: Correlation with portal pressure and variceal haemorrhage. Gastroenterology. 1989;96:873–80.
24. North Italian Endoscopic Club for the Study and Treatment of Oesophageal Varices. Prediction of the first variceal haemorrhage in patients with cirrhosis of the liver and oesophageal varices. N Engl J Med. 1988;319:983–9.
25. Pagliaro L, D'Amico G, Pasta L *et al.* Portal hypertension in cirrhosis: Natural history. In: Bosch J, Groszmann RJ, editors. Portal hypertension: Pathophysiology and treatment. Oxford, UK: Blackwell Scientific, 1994:72–92.
26. Violi F, Ferro D, Basili S *et al.* Hyperfibrinolysis increases the risk of gastrointestinal haemorrhage in patients with advanced cirrhosis. Hepatology. 1992;15:672–6.
27. Bomzon A. Vascular reactivity in liver disease. In: Blendis LM, Bomzon A, editors. Cardiovascular complications of liver disease. Boca Raton, FL: CRC Press, 1990:207–24.
28. Aldridge MC, Bismuth H. General surgical aspects and the risk of liver surgery in patients with hepatic disease. In: McIntyre N, Benhamou JP, Bircher J, Rizzetto M, Rodés J, editors. Oxford textbook of clinical hepatology. Oxford, UK: Oxford University Press, 1991:1403–10.
29. Graham DY, Smith JL. The course of patients after variceal haemorrhage. Gastroenterology. 1985;80:800–9.
30. Wood LJ, Colman J, Dudley FJ. The relationship between portal pressure and plasma albumin in the development of cirrhotic ascites. J Gastroenterol Hepatol. 1987;2:525–31.
31. Schrier RW, Arroyo V, Bernardi M, Epstein M, Henriksen JH, Rodés J. Peripheral arterial vasodilation hypothesis: A proposal for the initiation of renal sodium and water retention in cirrhosis. Hepatology. 1988;8:1151–8.
32. Blendis LM, Bomzon A. The cardiovascular complications of cirrhosis – A history. In: Blendis LM, Bomzon A, editors. Cardiovascular complications of liver disease. Boca Raton, FL: CRC Press, 1990:1–8.
33. Bernardi M, Trevisani F, Gasbarrini A, Gasbarrini G. Hepatorenal disorders: The role of renin–angiotensin–aldosterone system. Sem Liver Dis. 1994;14:23–34.
34. Arroyo V, Bosch J, Gaya J *et al.* Plasma renin activity and urinary sodium excretion as prognostic indicators in nonazotemic cirrhosis with ascites. Ann Intern Med. 1981;94:198–201.
35. Cosby RL, Yee B, Shrier RW. New classification with prognostic value in patients with cirrhosis. Minor Electrolyte Metab. 1988;15:261–6.
36. Runyon BA. Care of patients with ascites. N Engl J Med. 1994;330:337–42.
37. Runyon BA. Low-protein concentration ascitic fluid is predisposed to spontaneous bacterial peritonitis. Gastroenterology. 1986;91:1343–6.
38. Llach J, Rimola A, Navasa M *et al.* Incidence and predictive factors of first episode of spontaneous bacterial peritonitis in cirrhosis with ascites: Relevance of ascitic fluid protein concentration. Hepatology. 1992;16:724–7.
39. Pinzello G, Simonetti RG, Craxì A, Di Piazza S, Spanò S, Pagliaro L. Spontaneous bacterial peritonitis: A prospective investigation in predominantly non-alcoholic cirrhotic patients. Hepatology. 1983;3:545–9.
40. Kline M, McCallum R, Gruth PH. The clinical value of ascitic fluid culture and leukocyte count studies in alcoholic cirrhosis. Gastroenterology. 1976;70:408–12.
41. Pinzello G, Simonetti R, Cammà C *et al.* Spontaneous bacterial peritonitis: An update. Gastroenterol Int. 1993;6:54–60.
42. Llovet JM, Planas R, Morillas R *et al.* Short-term prognosis of cirrhotics with spontaneous bacterial peritonitis: Multivariate study. Am J Gastroenterol. 1993;88:388–92.
43. Runyon BA, McHutchinson JG, Antillon MR, Akriviadis EA, Montano AA. Short course versus long-course antibiotic treatment of spontaneous bacterial peritonitis. Gastroenterology. 1991;100:1737–42.
44. Titò L, Rimola A, Ginés P *et al.* Recurrence of spontaneous bacterial peritonitis in cirrhosis: Frequency and predictive factors. Hepatology. 1988;8:27–31.
45. Ginés P, Rimola A, Planas R *et al.* Norfloxacin prevents spontaneous bacterial peritonitis recurrence in cirrhosis: Results of a double-blind, placebo-controlled trial. Hepatology. 1990;12:716–24.

46. Soriano G, Guarner C, Teixido M *et al.* Selective intestinal decontamination prevents spontaneous bacterial peritonitis. Gastroenterology. 1991;100:477–81.
47. Agustì A, Roca J, Bosch J, Rodriguez-Roisin R. The lung in the liver disease. J Hepatol. 1990;10:251–7.
48. Rodés J, Bosch J, Arroyo V. Clinical types and drug therapy of renal impairment in cirrhosis. Postgrad Med J. 1975;51:492–7.
49. Runyon BA. Care of patients with ascites. N Engl J Med. 1994;330:337–42.
50. Ginés P, Arroyo V, Quintero E *et al.* Comparison of paracentesis and diuretics in the treatment of cirrhotics with tense ascites. Results of a randomized study. Gastroenterology. 1987;93:234–41.
51. Smart HL, Triger DR. A randomized prospective trial comparing daily paracentesis and intravenous albumin with recirculation in diuretic refractory ascites. J Hepatol. 1990;10:191–7.
52. Bernardi M, Rimondi A, Gasbarrini A *et al.* Ascites apheresis, concentration and reinfusion for the treatment of massive or refractory ascites in cirrhosis. J Hepatol. 1994;20:289–95.
53. Stanley MM, Ochi S, Lee KK *et al.* Peritoneovenous shunting as compared with medical treatment in patients with alcoholic cirrhosis and massive ascites. N Engl J Med. 1989;321:1632–8.
54. Ginés P, Arroyo V, Vargas V *et al.* Paracentesis with intravenous infusion of albumin as compared with peritoneovenous shunting in cirrhosis with refractory ascites. N Engl J Med. 1991;325:829–35.
55. Quiroga J, Sango B, Nunez M *et al.* Transjugular intrahepatic portal–systemic shunt in the treatment of refractory ascites: Effect on clinical, renal, humoral and hemodynamic parameters. Hepatology. 1995;21:986–94.
56. Lévy VG, Opolon P, Pauleau N, Caroli J. Treatment of ascites by reinfusion of concentrated peritoneal fluid – Review of 318 procedures in 210 patients. Postgrad Med J. 1975;51:564–6.
57. Epstein M. Peritoneovenous shunt in the management of ascites and hepatorenal syndrome. Gastroenterology. 1982;82:790–9.
58. Rössle M, Ochs A, Haag K. TIPS: Problem and clinical results. In: Holstege A, Schölmerich J, Hahn EG, editors. Portal hypertension. Lancaster, UK: Kluwer Academic, 1995:328–34.
59. Bernardi M, Trevisani F. Cirrhosis with ascites: A heterogeneous population. Hepatology. 1987;7:199–200.
60. Bernardi M, Trevisani F, Gasbarrini G. The renin–angiotensin–aldosterone system in liver disease. In: Bomzon A, Blendis AM, editors. Cardiovascular complications of liver disease. Boca Raton FL: CRC Press, 1990:29–62.
61. Bernardi M, Trevisani F, De Palma R *et al.* Chronobiological evaluation of sympathoadrenergic function in cirrhosis. Relationship with arterial pressure and heart rate. Gastroenterology. 1987;93:1178–86.
62. Arroyo V, Epstein M, Gallus G, Gentilini P, Ring-Larsen H, Salerno F. Refractory ascites in cirrhosis: Mechanism and treatment. Gastroenterol Int. 1989;2:195–207.
63. Pagliaro L, Simonetti RG. Ascite: storia naturale e trattamento. BIMS. 1995;56:4–18.
64. Ginés A, Escorsell A, Ginés P *et al.* Incidence, predictive factors, and prognosis of the hepatorenal syndrome in cirrhosis with ascites. Gastroenterology. 1993;105:229–36.
65. Epstein M. Hepatorenal syndrome. In: Epstein M, editor. The kidney in liver disease (3rd edition). Baltimore: Williams and Wilkins, 1988;89–118.
66. Cuervas-Mons V, Millan I, Gavaler JS, Starzl TE, Van Thiel DH. Prognostic value of preoperatively obtained clinical and laboratory data in predicting survival following orthotopic liver transplantation. Hepatology. 1986;6:922–7.
67. Rimola A, Gavaler JS, Schade RR, El-Lankany S, Starzl T, Van Thiel DH. Effects of renal impairment on liver transplantation. Gastroenterology. 1987;93:148–56.
68. Haagsma BH, Gips CH, Wesenhagen H *et al.* Liver disease and its effect on hemostasis during liver transplantation. Liver. 1985;5:123–8.
69. Titò L, Ginés P, Arroyo V *et al.* Total paracentesis with intravenous albumin in the management of patients with cirrhosis and ascites. Gastroenterology. 1990;98:146–51.
70. Planas R, Ginés P, Arroyo V *et al.* Dextran-70 versus albumin as plasma expanders in cirrhotic patients with tense ascites treated with total paracentesis. Results of a randomized study. Gastroenterology. 1990;99:1736–44.
71. Salerno F, Badalamenti S, Lorenzano E, Moser P, Incerti P. Randomized comparative study of hemaccel vs. albumin infusion after total paracentesis in cirrhotic patients with refractory ascites. Hepatology. 1991;13:707–13.

72. Ginés A, Planas R, Angeli P *et al.* Treatment of patients with cirrhosis and refractory ascites using LeVeen shunt with Titanium tip: Comparison with therapeutic paracentesis. Hepatology. 1995;22:124–31.
73. Ratnoff OD, Patek AJ Jr. The natural history of Laennec's cirrhosis of the liver; analysis of 386 cases. Medicine (Baltimore). 1942;21:207–68.
74. Castells A, Salò J, Planas R *et al.* Impact of shunt surgery for variceal bleeding in the natural history of ascites in cirrhosis: A retrospective study. Hepatology. 1994;20:584–91.

Section IV
New and Old Markers

12 Serum markers for liver fibrosis – current and future developments

D. SCHUPPAN, T. AKSÜ, P. LIBUDA, C. KOSZKA and H. HERBST

MECHANISMS OF LIVER FIBROSIS

Repeated parenchymal cell damage underlies all chronic liver diseases. It paves the way for fibrosis and finally cirrhosis. Usually, damage or necrosis of hepatocytes or bile duct epithelia, e.g. by hepatotoxins or a T-cell response to virus-bearing or otherwise altered parenchymal cells, causes activation of mononuclear cells that release fibrogenic factors which induce proliferation and collagen synthesis of liver mesenchymal cells[1–4]. Whereas activated Kupffer cells and macrophages are the primary sources of fibrogenic cytokines and growth factors[1–6], hepatic stellate cells (synonyms: perisinusoidal lipocytes, Ito cells) and portal fibroblasts have been identified as the central collagen producing cells in the liver[1–7]. Similar cells are also implicated in fibrosis of other organs such as kidney (mesangial cells and interstitial fibroblasts), lung (alveolar and interstitial fibroblasts), intestine and arteries[8–10]. After activation, these usually quiescent cells undergo transformation into a myofibroblastic phenotype characterized by a high rate of proliferation and the production of excess collagen. As shown in Figure 1, these myofibroblast-like cells can secrete fibrogenic growth factors themselves, thus maintaining an autocrine and paracrine loop of activation. As in other organs, the fibroproliferative response of the liver is aimed at a rapid wound closure and subsides if the offending agent is only present for a limited period of time. However, after repeated damage to the liver, the expansion of the mesenchymal compartment may be self-sustaining due to the vicious circle of autocrine stimulation mentioned above, even in the absence of overt necrosis or inflammation. Therefore, strategies must be designed that halt the progression of liver fibrosis or even reverse cirrhosis. Targets for antifibrotic therapy are the fibrogenic cell types, the fibrogenic growth factors or their cellular sources.

THE HEPATIC EXTRACELLULAR MATRIX

The (collagenous) extracellular matrix (ECM) was originally considered a metabolically inert material that merely served as a structural framework for the

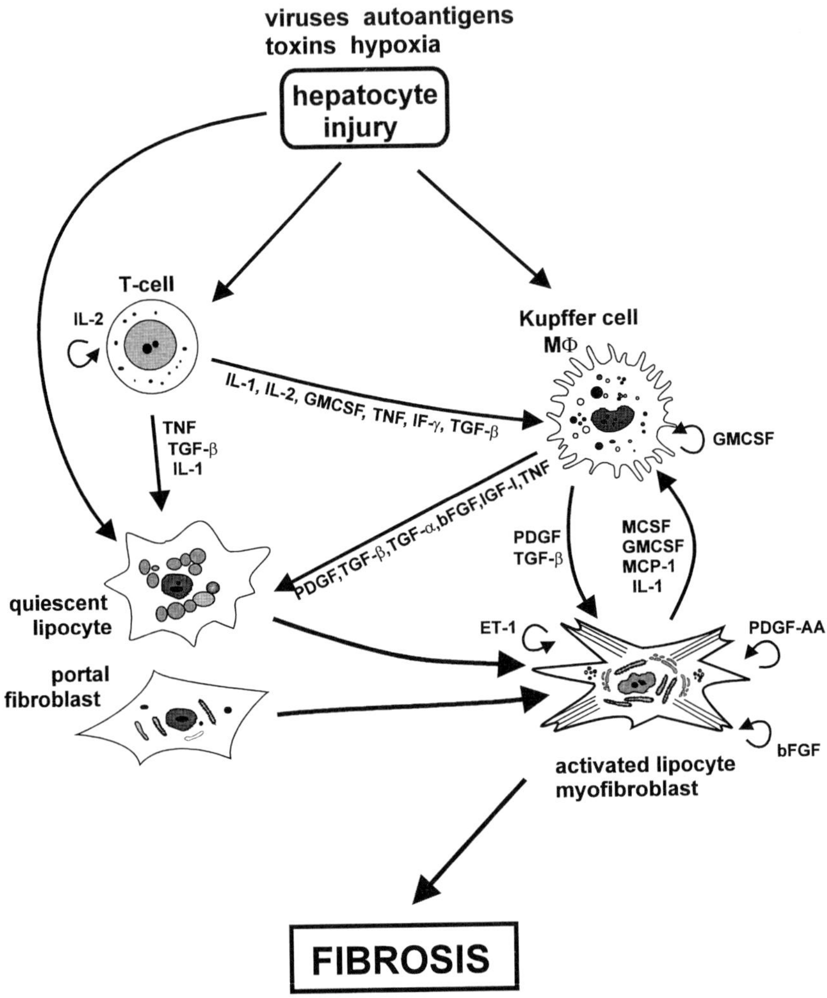

Fig. 1 Mechanisms of liver fibrogenesis. In liver as well as in other organs prone to fibrosis, a usually quiescent mesenchymal cell such as the portal fibroblast and the hepatic stellate cell (perisinusoidal lipocyte) is activated to transform into a myofibroblastic phenotype with numerous actin stress fibres, a hypertrophied rough endoplasmic reticulum, high rate of proliferation and a potential to synthesize large amounts of collagen. Other cell types such as sinusoidal endothelial cells (which are important for angiogenesis and, once damaged, secrete fibrogenic factors), activated platelets (which release fibrogenic factors like PDGF and TGF-β) and granulocytes (which produce reactive oxygen species that lead to the release of cytokines from neighbouring cells) are also involved in the pathogenesis of liver fibrosis, but not shown. IL, interleukin; TNF, tumour necrosis factor; (G)MCSF, (granulocyte) macrophage colony stimulating factor; IF, interferon; TGF, transforming growth factor; PDGF, platelet-derived growth factor; bFGF, basic fibroblast growth factor; MCP, macrophage chemotactic peptide; ET, endothelin (from reference 4, with permission)

functionally important parenchyma. On the contrary, the liver ECM, like the ECM of other epithelial–mesenchymal organs, is a complex assembly of macromolecules that once injured, rapidly undergoes remodelling, in order to re-establish cellular functions and tissue homeostasis. Accordingly, the macromolecules of the ECM provide resident and immigrating (e.g. inflammatory) cells with spatial signals that are indispensable for migration, proliferation, differentiation or for the establishment of cell polarity[3,11]. The regulatory role of the ECM is underlined by the characterization of cellular receptors for ECM proteins (mainly the integrins) that can modulate classical intracellular signal transduction pathways. Classically, the molecules of the ECM have been subdivided into collagens, non-collagenous glycoproteins, glycosaminoglycans, proteoglycans and elastin[1,3,12–14]. But many ECM molecules are in fact hybrids with structural and functional properties characteristic for different classes, such as collagen XIV that contains more than 90% of non-collagenous sequences and only a short collagenous tail. In an extended view, other molecules that regularly or occasionally associate with the classical ECM components should also be included as ECM constituents. Examples are ECM degrading matrix metalloproteinases (MMPs) and their inhibitors, the tissue inhibitors of metalloproteinases (TIMPs)[15,16] and a variety of growth factors and cytokines. Binding of growth factors by certain matrix molecules leads to their storage in a matrix-dependent pattern and to modulation of their biological activities[3,14,17,18] (Figure 2). Once released by matrix degrading enzymes such as the MMPs, these factors can initiate cell proliferation, angiogensis and ECM deposition, processes that are directed at the restitution of organ homeostasis.

ANTIFIBROTIC TREATMENT

Several studies have shown that *interferons*, with interferon-γ being more potent than interferons-α and -β, can suppress collagen synthesis *in vitro* and *in vivo*[19–21]. Interferons suppress the spontaneous activation of rat hepatic lipocytes, and decrease the expression of procollagen and fibronectin mRNAs to between 3 and 24% of controls, whereas total protein synthesis and cell survival are almost unaffected[22].

Prostaglandins E (PGE) decrease the hepatic collagen content in rat models of liver fibrosis either induced by nutrient deficiency[23] or following bile duct ligation and scission[24]. PGE causes a down regulation of procollagen mRNA expression in lipocytes, perhaps via an increase of intracellular cAMP. Similarly, *relaxin*, a hormone that initiates uterine involution by decreasing collagen synthesis and enhancing the activity of interstitial collagenase, induces the autocrine and paracrine synthesis of PGE. When injected together with interferon-γ, relaxin prevents collagen deposition in experimental granulation tissue[25].

Other so-called hepatotropic and hepatoprotective drugs that have minimal side-effects and that can be administered by the oral route have been rediscovered as potential antifibrotic agents. Dilinoleyl-phosphatidyl-choline, the active compound of *polyunsaturated lecithin* (PUL), has prevented severe fibrosis and cirrhosis in baboons fed a diet containing 50% ethanol[26]. The pro-

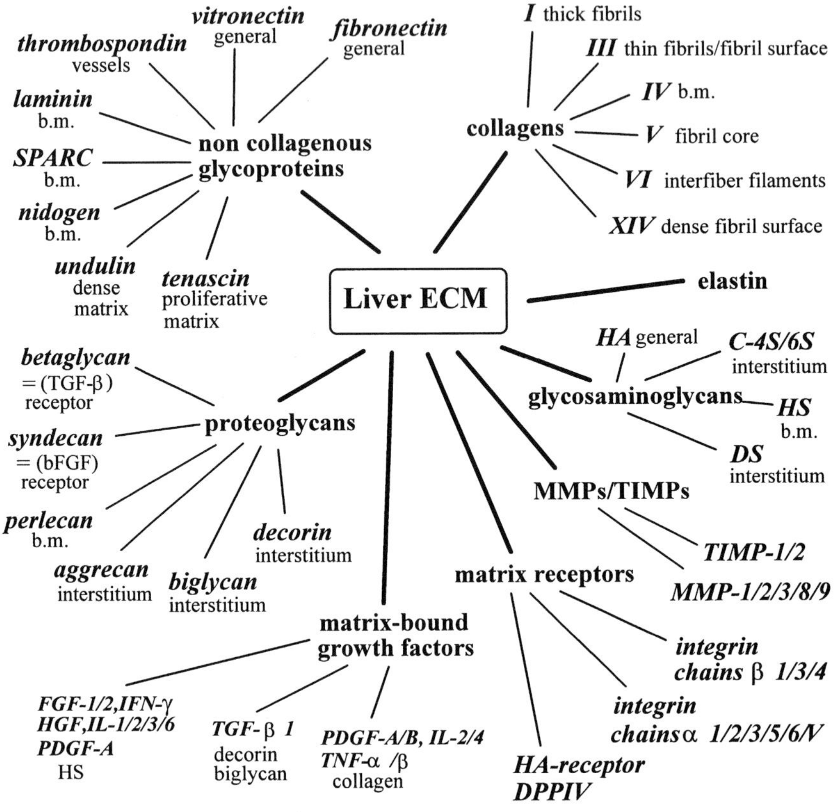

Fig. 2 The hepatic extracellular matrix. Overview of the collagen types, non-collagenous glycoproteins, elastin, glycosaminoglycans and proteoglycans that have been found in the liver ECM. The matrix-bound growth factors/cytokines, metalloproteinases (MMPs), tissue inhibitors of metalloproteinases (TIMPs) and integrins have been included, since they can specifically associate with the ECM. SPARC, secreted protein acidic and rich in cysteine (synonymous with osteonectin or BM-40); b.m., basement membrane; HA, hyaluronic acid; C-4S/6S, chondroitin 4/6-sulfate; HS, heparan sulfate; DS, dermatan sulfate; DPPIV, dipeptidyl peptidase IV (from reference 14, with permission)

posed mechanism is a stimulation of collagenase activity in rat hepatic stellate cells irrespective of the presence or the absence of the toxic metabolite acetaldehyde[27].

Similarly, *silymarin*, a standardized phytopharmacon with the polyphenole silibinin as the major active ingredient, has reduced collagen accumulation in rat secondary biliary fibrosis[28]. The antifibrotic effects of both PUL and silymarin are currently being addressed by large multicentre clinical trials that include patients with alcoholic liver fibrosis and cirrhosis. Furthermore, it has been shown that *ursodeoxycholic acid* can decrease fibrogenesis and increase fibrolysis in rat secondary biliary fibrosis[29] and, by using surrogate markers of liver fibrosis (see below), in patients with primary biliary cirrhosis[30].

Other drugs for which an antifibrotic potential could be demonstrated in suitable rat models of liver fibrosis include *retinoids*[31] and *pentoxifylline*[32], whereas drug-targeting of the prolyl 4-hydroxylase inhibitors that prevent the production of stable collagen triple helices[33] has to be improved. The latter agents are specifically activated in hepatocytes, but it is unclear if they reach the fibrogenic cells (i.e. the hepatic stellate cells and the portal fibroblasts).

Intensive research is aimed at the neutralization or localized removal of fibrogenic growth factors. An example is transforming growth factor $\beta 1$ (TGF-$\beta 1$), a key fibrogenic factor that enhances ECM deposition and inhibits collagenase activities[34]. Experimental kidney fibrosis could be prevented by the i.v. injection of recombinant decorin, a small extracellular proteoglycan that can bind and sequester TGF-$\beta 1$ in the ECM[35]. Similarly, platelet-derived growth factor (PDGF), a potent mitogen for hepatic stellate cells[36], is bound to liver collagens at sites of excessive release. Since this interaction is mediated by a collagenous consensus sequence, peptide analogues can be designed that remove the excess PDGF deposited in the ECM[37]. Efforts also focus on the design of receptor antagonists for TGF-$\beta 1$ and PDGF, either in the form of recombinant extracellular receptor domains or synthetic non-peptidic inhibitors (unpublished data).

Further in this line, certain peptides or their non-peptidic analogues which are derived from ECM molecules and which serve as recognition sequences for matrix receptors could become future antifibrotic agents. Thus derivatives of the tripeptide Arg-Gly-Asp inhibit the interaction of various integrins (ECM-receptors) with the ECM and can induce stress relaxation of fibrogenic cells, a process that is associated with a decrease in collagen synthesis and an increase in collagenases[38]. Stress relaxation also mitigates signals transferred via the receptors for PDGF and other mitogenic growth factors[39], which is due to the necessity of integrin-mediated signals from the ECM for growth factor-induced signal transduction[11]. Great effort is currently being spent on the identification of more potent and more specific ECM peptides[40,41], and in the development of biologically stable non-peptidic analogues[42] that modulate cell behaviour and induce stress-relaxation. Current and future antifibrotic strategies are summarized in Figure 3.

SELECTION OF SUITABLE ANIMAL MODELS OF LIVER FIBROSIS

The selection of suitable experimental models that are as close as possible to the human disease is of primary importance, both in studies of the pathobiochemistry of liver fibrosis and for the testing of potential antifibrotic agents[43,44]. Preclinical testing of such agents in appropriate *in vivo* models, preferably in rats, is indispensible, since animals can be sacrificed at certain time points, and total hepatic collagen, the gold standard for antifibrotic therapy, can be determined in untreated vs. treated groups. Unfortunately, most rat models that were used in the past were based on hepatotoxins such as carbon tetrachloride, thioacetamide or N-dimethyl-nitrosamine. These chemicals give rise to free radicals that cause centroacinar or panlobular hepatocyte necrosis and regeneration[43–45]. Although repeated application of the toxins can induce fibrosis

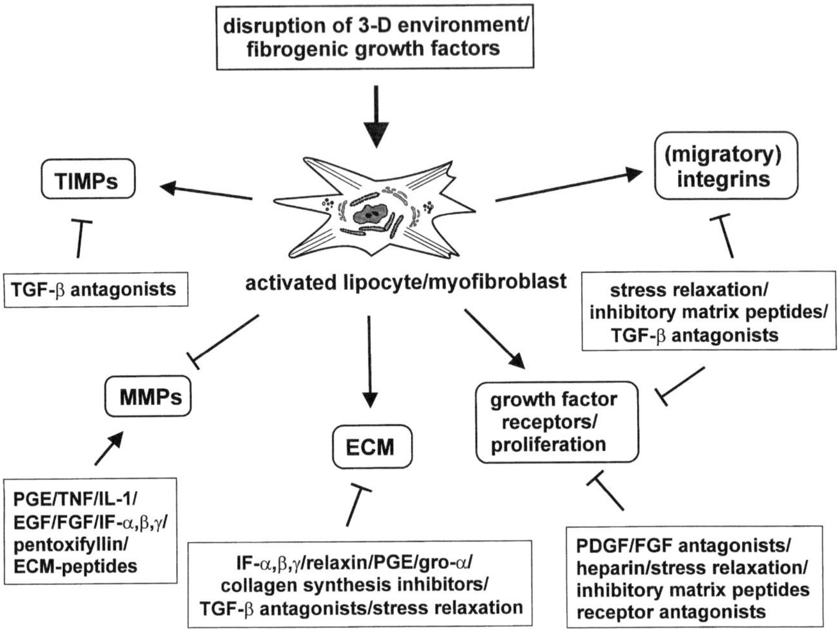

Fig. 3 Antifibrotic strategies. Several strategies to inhibit liver fibrogenesis appear feasible. These strategies may be targeted at stress-inducing integrins, fibrogenic growth factors and their receptors, the genes that regulate collagen synthesis or at the tissue inhibitors (TIMPs) of matrix metalloproteinases (MMPs). Alternatively, certain agents could be used to enhance the expression and activity of MMPs, especially MMP-1, which is down-regulated in the fibrogenic cells. Whereas many of these approaches may have potential to induce systemic side-effects, some strategies, such as the inhibition of fibrogenic growth factor activities at the site of their major production and deposition, and the use of biologically stable non-peptidic analogues of bioactive ECM-peptides that modulate integrins and stress signals, hold promise for the future (from reference 4, with permission)

and finally cirrhosis, the models do not allow validation of potential antifibrotic drugs, since anti-inflammatory and radical-scavenging properties cannot be differentiated from a true antifibrotic effect. Although inflammation and free radicals initiate and exacerbate most liver diseases, as exemplified in viral hepatitis and alcoholic hepatitis, they often play a minor role in the progression of fibrosis in chronic conditions. As an example, immunosuppressants and radical scavengers do not prevent or even retard fibrosis in human chronic hepatitis. Therefore, only models that are not based on radical-mediated hepatocyte damage and that are devoid of massive inflammation and necrosis, such as rat biliary fibrosis secondary to occlusion or scission of the common bile duct, should be considered. This model produces a progressive portal fibrosis and finally cirrhosis, with an up to tenfold increased collagen content in the liver[46]. Furthermore, the availability of several serum markers of liver fibrosis for rat as well as man, promises to speed-up their validation as parameters of prognosis and antifibrotic therapy control in clinical studies (see below).

NECESSITY FOR SERUM MARKERS OF LIVER FIBROSIS

Since liver fibrosis and cirrhosis in man usually develop over many years, frequent follow-up biopsies are not suitable for monitoring histological progression. Furthermore, there is always an uncertainty of sampling error caused by focal differences of inflammation and fibrosis, a characteristic of most liver diseases[47], and finally, frequent biopsies are both ethically and practically unacceptable. Therefore, serum markers of liver fibrosis that can be determined on a day-to-day basis and that allow a non-invasive and rapid assessment of *de novo* collagen deposition, i.e. *fibrogenesis*, and *de novo* collagen removal, i.e. *fibrolysis*, in the liver, are urgently needed. Such assays could yield prognostic information as to the propensity of a patient to progress to cirrhosis and enable the clinician to decide within a few days or weeks, if the patient should be given a potential antifibrotic agent over a long term. In addition, serum tests should reflect the dynamics of fibrogenesis and fibrolysis in the *whole liver*, information that can never be provided by a tiny biopsy. It can be anticipated that, once certain parameters of liver fibrosis have been validated as prognostic markers of fibrogenesis or fibrolysis, the discovery and clinical utilization of antifibrotic drugs will grow exponentially.

PROPERTIES OF AN IDEAL MARKER

Ideally, serum assays for liver fibrosis should fulfil several requirements. They should:

1. be specific for the liver, with no major contribution by other organs;
2. be sensitive enough to detect minor changes of fibrogenesis and fibrolysis;
3. reflect either fibrogenesis, fibrolysis or the amount of connective tissue laid down in the liver, and not merely an enhanced connective tissue turnover;
4. have a known biological half-life and known major routes of disposal and excretion, in order to allow a better interpretation of changing serum levels and the role of, for example, reduced kidney or liver function;
5. derive from a defined cellular source in the diseased liver, preferably the activated mesenchymal cells, and not hepatocytes, in order to exclude, for example, interference by a functionally and synthetically compromised parenchyma;
6. be measurable by sensitive, rapid and easy-to-perform assay formats, such as the ELISA technique, that do not require expensive equipment or a nuclear medicine department; and
7. be standardized and validated by reference laboratories, to ensure comparability of results.

VALIDITY OF CURRENT MARKERS

As is the case with most clinical chemical parameters, the available serum markers for liver fibrosis do not come up to the requirements of ideal parameters[13,14,48,49]. However, biochemical, animal experimental and clinical studies of the last few years have provided numerous data that permit a preliminary assessment of how far certain markers mirror fibrogenesis and/or fibrolysis in the liver.

Fortunately, most of the measurable connective tissue antigens show the highest levels in active liver diseases, with only minor contributions by other systemic inflammatory or fibrotic conditions such as pulmonary fibrosis, rheumatoid arthritis and the so-called 'collagen diseases'[50,51]. Similarly, serum levels are only slightly influenced by localized fibrogenesis as in pulmonary fibrosis or wound healing after major surgery for example[52,53]. However, circulating fibrosis markers may be increased up to two- or threefold in chronic renal diseases that are associated with kidney fibrosis. This has been shown for *PIIINP* (the aminoterminal propeptide of procollagen III), *PIVCP* (the carboxyterminal propeptide of procollagen IV), *collagen VI* and *undulin*[54–56]. Unexpectedly though, the kidney does not appear to play a significant role in the elimination of these antigens, since their clearance remains low and does not change significantly with progressive functional renal impairment. Similarly, these markers do not correlate with serum creatinine or creatinine clearance, suggesting that the fibrotic kidney itself can be an important contributor to increased serum levels. Other conditions that may cause increased levels of fibrosis markers such as bulky tumours, especially those with metastasis to the liver, can usually be excluded by clinical assessment[48,57].

When selecting assays for liver fibrosis, one has to consider the distribution and occurrence of the target antigen. An example is collagen/procollagen I, the major ECM protein of liver. Although assays exist for several of its structural domains, namely the N- and C-terminal propeptides, the telopeptides and the helical portion, their usefulness for the assessment of liver diseases is limited due to interference by a dominating bone metabolism[58–60].

A major problem for the interpretation of raised serum levels of a given marker is the heterogeneity of circulating antigens usually encountered. Analysis of this is commonly performed by subjecting normal and pathological sera to molecular sieve chromatography and quantitation of immunoreactive material in the fractions eluted. In this regard, PIIINP-immunoreactivity in normal serum elutes as four major peaks, with the intact aminopropeptide of Mr 50 kD as a minor species, with a prominent peak of its degradation product, fragment Col 1 of Mr 10 kD, and two fractions of higher Mr, probably representing dimeric propeptide and propeptide linked to the collagen helix[48]. In active liver disease, the proportion of the intact propeptide of Mr 50 kD may increase relative to the other fractions. Only the propeptide that is released in stoichiometric amounts when newly secreted procollagen III is incorporated into the growing collagen fibril can be attributed to fibrogenesis, whereas the other fragments might also derive from the degradation of preexisting fibrils. This ambiguity results from the retention of a partially processed form of procollagen III that contains the aminopropeptide still covalently attached to the collagen helix which forms a surface coat on the resting fibril[13,14,48]. This problem has in part been circumvented by the introduction of novel assays that detect the molecular species which contain PIIINP and not the less antigenic but quantitatively predominant fragment Col 1 (Behring RIAgnost, Pharmacia PIIIP).

Circulating antigens that, due to their high molecular weight, can be related both to fibrogenesis and fibrolysis have been found for *basement membrane collagen* and for *laminin*, the major non-collagenous glycoprotein of basement membranes[61,62]. Because these antigens are not cleaved off during matrix assembly, contrary to the above discussed PIIINP, they should rather result from fibrolysis and enhanced basement membrane turnover. The observed correlation of the basement membrane markers with the degree of liver fibrosis[61–68], can perhaps be explained by the progressive sinusoidal capillarization and the vascular proliferations that accompany the enlargement of portal fields.

The finding that 80–90% of serum *collagen VI* and *undulin*, two large proteins of the interstitial ECM that also lack propeptide segments, are of low molecular weight, clearly assigns them a role as markers of fibrolysis (reviewed in[13,14]). Although the kidneys[54–56] and the biliary system[69] appear to be minor routes of excretion of circulating connective tissue molecules, the outstanding role of liver sinusoidal endothelial cells in their receptor-mediated uptake and perhaps degradation, adds further complexity to the matter, potentially reducing the markers to mere parameters of liver blood flow and endothelial cell function. Thus it has been shown that hyaluronic acid, a polyglycan of most connective tissues, is cleared from blood with a half-life of only a few minutes[70,71], qualifying it rather as an indicator of sinusoidal endothelial function than of connective tissue turnover.

Similarly, PIIINP[72], the propeptides of procollagen I[73] and the basement membrane proteins laminin and nidogen[74] have been shown to be cleared by sinusoidal endothelial cells. However, the disappearance of radioactively-labelled PIIINP from serum, as recently determined in the normal pig, follows a two-order kinetics with half lives of about 45 minutes and 8 hours[75]. These data are in accord with previous findings published in abstract form[76] that showed that PIIINP and PIVCP (synonymous with NC1, the C-terminal fragment of procollagen IV) have serum half-lives of approximately 25 minutes and 6–10 hours in normal rats. These half-lives were not changed (PIIINP) or even shortened (PIVCP) in rats with secondary biliary fibrosis, although the initial uptake in the normal liver, which for PIIINP reached 86% of the injected radioactivity within 3–7 minutes, was retarded and reduced to approximately 60% in cirrhotic animals. Therefore, it may be tentatively concluded that a reduction in liver perfusion and function do not result in an increase of PIIINP and PIVCP serum levels. That this might apply to other markers seems possible but awaits future demonstration.

Table 1 lists the serum markers that have been studied in man and/or rat and their preliminary assignment to either fibrogenesis, fibrolysis or both.

EXPERIMENTAL AND CLINICAL VALIDATION OF THE MARKERS

As mentioned above, increased levels of *PIIINP* may reflect fibrogenesis during continuous fibril growth as well as a sudden bout of fibrolysis from already deposited collagen. This explains why PIIINP alone appears to be of little prognostic value in acute conditions such as acute viral or alcoholic hepatitis, where inflammation, consecutive matrix degradation and matrix synthesis coexist. But there is now plenty of information indicating that in chronic progressive liver diseases, PIIINP can be used as a parameter of fibrogenesis.

Table 1 Serum assays for liver fibrosis

	Fibrogenesis	*Fibrolysis*	*'Liver specificity'*
PICP	+	–	(+), *bone*
PIIINP	+	(+), *acute*	+
PIVCP	– (?)	+	+ (*fibrosis*)
PIVNP	– (?)	+	+ (*fibrosis*)
Hyaluronan	+ (?)	+ (?)	(+) (*fibrosis*)
Laminin	+ (?)	+ (?)	(+) (*fibrosis*)
Collagen VI	–	+	(+)
Undulin	–	+ (*portal*)	+
Tenascin	+ (*lobular*)	–	+ (?)
TIMP-1	+	–	+ (?)
Collagenase I	–	+	+ (?)
Integrin $\beta 1$	+	(+)	(+)
Integrin α chains	+	(+)	+ (?) (*proliferation*)
TGF-$\beta 1$	+	–	+ (?)

PICP, C-terminal propeptide of procollagen I; PIIINP, N-terminal propeptide of procollagen III; PIVCP, C-terminal propeptide of procollagen IV (NC1-fragment); PIVNP, N-terminal propeptide of procollagen IV (7-S collagen); TIMP-1, tissue inhibitor of metalloproteinases 1; TGF-$\beta 1$, transforming growth factor beta. Data on TGF-$\beta 1$ and integrin α chains (own unpublished results) are preliminary. 'Liver specificity' denotes that most marked elevations are observed in liver diseases. PIIINP may reflect fibrolysis in acute bouts of hepatitis. For further details refer to the text

One line of evidence comes from rat experimental studies using models characterized by progressive fibrosis and little inflammation or necrosis, such as a nutrient deficient diet and biliary fibrosis secondary to obliteration of the common bile duct[23,46]. In these models, sequential measurement of PIIINP, i.e. PIIINP levels integrated over time, correctly predicted the amount of collagen that accumulated in the livers. Accordingly, a decreased PIIINP allowed an early assessment of the antifibrotic potential of prostaglandin-derivatives in the model of nutrient deficiency[23].

PIIINP also correlated with total collagen accumulation and its inhibition in rats with secondary biliary fibrosis that were treated with the drugs silymarin and pentoxifyllin[28,32]. Furthermore, PIIINP predicted mRNA levels for liver procollagen type III in the pre-cirrhotic phase of carbon tetrachloride-induced fibrosis[77].

Studies in man showed that enhanced PIIINP indicated an increase in bioactive liver prolyl hydroxylase, a key enzyme for synthesis of stable collagen[78]. In patients with chronic viral hepatitis subjected to treatment with interferon, serum PIIINP correlated well with the mRNA encoding liver procollagen $\alpha 1$(I) and of the fibrogenic mediater TGF-$\beta 1$, but not with AST, a surrogate marker of inflammatory activity[20]. These more recent findings shed novel light on earlier studies performed in a follow-up design that demonstrated that PIIINP may be of great value in predicting the development of chronic active vs. chronic persistent hepatitis when other serological parameters fail[79–84], whereas the suggestion of PIIINP as a strong and independent predictor of the natural evolution of primary biliary cirrhosis[85,86] has been challenged by others[87].

As already mentioned, the data generated in earlier studies have to be interpreted with caution, since assay variants with differing sensitivities for the antigenic species related to PIIINP were used. The former non-equilibrium RIA mainly detected antigenically intact PIIINP[79], the RIA using Fab antibody fragments measured intact PIIINP as well as the Col 1 antigen resulting from degradation of collagen fibrils to a similar degree[88], and the older coated tube variant (RIAgnost) picked up a significant portion of Col 1 in addition to PIIINP.

More recent assays, namely the already mentioned equilibrium RIA based on human PIIINP[89] and an improved RIAgnost system that do not react with the Col 1 fragment are now commercially available, promising more reliable and better standardized versions of this surrogate marker of fibrogenesis. PIIINP has been increasingly used in follow-up studies of patients with hepatitis C, and to a minor degree hepatitis B, who were treated with interferon-α. Most groups reported a normalization of PIIINP in complete responders[90–94]. Interestingly, three of these studies also reported a fall of PIIINP in interferon-treated patients who showed no or only a partial response[90,92,94]. Since PIIINP remained suppressed in the latter patients, even 12 months after interferon was stopped, the agent might have a prolonged antifibrogenic effect that is independent of the serological response and decrease of necroinflammation. This assumption is further supported by histological follow-up studies that suggest a decrease of the amount of hepatic collagen, irrespective of the clinical and serological response to interferon[21,95].

In search for a marker of interstitial collagen degradation, we found that circulating *collagen VI*, a molecule that runs in filaments between large collagen fibrils, is a mixture of low molecular weight fragments, characterizing it as a marker of fibrolysis[60,96]. Since both collagen VI and PIIINP derive from similar sites in the interstitial ECM, their simultaneous measurement in a patient could allow an assessment of the balance between fibrogenesis and fibrolysis. In this line, most but not all patients with primary biliary cirrhosis stage I-IV, who had been treated with ursodeoxycholic acid for 2–4 years, showed a decrease of PIIINP and an increase of collagen VI, indicating a favourable course in terms of the progression of fibrosis[30]. In addition, serum collagen VI is not increased in young children, whereas other fibrosis markers, especially PIIINP, and to a minor degree, basement membrane related antigens, are not well suited to monitoring liver disease in this age group due to elevated levels that are related to body growth[97,98]. In small children serum collagen VI allowed detection of chronic fibrotic liver disease with a sensitivity and specificity of almost 100%[99]. But generalized connective tissue diseases and renal fibrosis, that can lead to elevated collagen VI levels, have to be excluded[13,14,56].

Undulin is a glycoprotein related to collagen XIV. It associates with the surface of mature fibrillar collagen[100] in the dense interstitial ECM, and appears to be removed rapidly when the normal collagen architecture is disturbed. Thus it is not surprising that serum undulin increases 3–5 fold even in early stages of alcoholic liver disease, of schistosomiasis and of primary biliary cirrhosis when markers like PIIINP are in the normal range[101,102]. Since, as for collagen VI, the detected antigens derive from fibrolysis, serum undulin is now included in several clinical studies with potential antifibrotic drugs.

Data concerning the polyglycan *hyaluronic acid* are still somewhat controversial. Although it is now established that its serum levels increase with the progression of fibrosis[68,103–107], the broad ranges of hyaluronic acid values in the groups of patients with a given stage of fibrosis, coupled with its rapid and high uptake by sinusoidal endothelial cells (see above), may make it a less suitable serum marker.

A serum test for the $\beta1$ chain of *integrins* has been added to the spectrum of assayable fibrosis markers[108]. Integrins are receptors for molecules of the ECM or function as cell–cell adhesion molecules[3,11,109]. Most of the integrin matrix receptors are composed of a common $\beta1$ chain that forms a heterodimer with an α-chain, and the α-chain defines the substrate specificity. Since essentially all cell types of the body bear a spectrum of $\beta1$ integrins on their surface, an increase of the serum $\beta1$ chain can be anticipated in multiple conditions of inflammation, fibrosis and cell death. Accordingly, this parameter, which correlates with hepatic inflammation, necrosis and fibrosis, shows little specificity[108].

Tenascin, a non-collagenous glycoprotein, is absent from the portal tract stroma but found in the perisinusoidal space of normal liver. It is highly expressed *de novo* in periportal zones, around vascular and bile ductular proliferations and in the space of Disse during active fibrogenesis, whereas it is rapidly removed when a metabolically quiescent scar is formed[110]. In a cross-sectional study, serum tenascin has been found elevated in patients with acute and chronic liver diseases, but it was not judged superior to other fibrosis markers in the diagnosis of fibrosis and cirrhosis[111]. However, by using a different assay, tenascin was decreased by 50% in all our patients with chronic hepatitis B and C during and up to 6 months after interferon treatment, with comparable values for responders and non-responders, whereas it was in the normal range in 22 patients with primary biliary cirrhosis stage I–IV[112]. This led us to conclude that tenascin could be a selective marker of sinusoidal fibrogenesis that adds a novel dimension to the non-invasive assessment of local aspects of fibrogenesis in the liver.

Circulating *collagenases* or their activities are of interest, since biochemical[113] as well as *in situ* hybridization studies[114] have demonstrated that the activity and expression of the enzyme that degrades fibrillar collagen I (interstitial collagenase, matrix metalloproteinase 1, MMP-1) wanes with progression to advanced fibrosis. Recently, circulating collagen I degrading activity was determined enzymatically in patients with chronic liver diseases and found to be inversely correlated with serum PIIINP[115], suggesting that mechanisms that suppress collagenase activity and expression are operative during active fibrogenesis. In addition, *in situ* hybridization demonstrated a high-level expression of *TIMP-1* (tissue inhibitor of metalloproteinase 1), the most potent natural inhibitor of MMP-1, in hepatic stellate cells and occasional hepatocytes in areas of active fibrogenesis[116]. *TIMP-1* can now been measured in serum, and a study showed it to be a sensitive marker of incipient alcoholic liver fibrosis[117]. Since only one other, cross-sectional investigation of patients with chronic viral hepatitis has been performed, in which TIMP-1 was correlated to histological scores of fibrosis and inflammation[68], follow-up studies are needed for further evaluation.

FUTURE DIRECTIONS

The important question that arises from the experiences of the past and present is: how can we make sure that the fibrosis markers that we are using are truly predicting fibrogenesis, fibrolysis or the early remodelling of liver ECM? To ensure progress in this field, future research has to focus on several aspects:

1. More follow-up studies have to be designed that apply improved scores of histological fibrosis.
2. There is a need for studies performing quantitative reverse transcription polymerase chain reaction (RT-PCR) from liver biopsy material, quantifying mRNA levels for, for example, procollagens I and III, MMP-1 and TGF-β1, which are expected to correlate with circulating fibrosis markers. Although the development of a quantitative RT-PCR from tiny biopsies is fraught with problems, a cooperative approach at the European level in this direction is already underway.
3. Potential antifibrotic agents should be tested in suitable rat models of liver fibrosis; in these models serum markers like PIIINP that are also available for man should be measured as early predictors of therapy response.
4. Markers with higher and novel specificities must be developed.
5. More rapid, more easy-to-perform and more specific assay formats that allow 'beside analysis' should be designed.

Acknowledgements

Part of the authors' own studies were supported by grants Schu 646/1-1/4 and SFB 366 C5 from Deutsche Forschungsgemeinschaft. D.S. is recipient of a Hermann-und-Lilly-Schilling-professorship.

References

1. Gressner AM. Hepatic fibrogenesis: The puzzle of interacting cells, fibrogenic cytokines, regulatory loops, and extracellular matrix molecules. Z Gastroenterol (S1). 1992;30:5–16.
2. Friedman SL. The cellular basis of hepatic fibrosis. N Engl J Med. 1993;328:1826–35.
3. Schuppan D, Herbst H, Milani S. Matrix, matrix synthesis and molecular networks in hepatic fibrosis. In: Zern MA, Reid L, editors. Extracellular matrix. Chemistry, biology and pathobiology with emphasis on the liver. New York: Marcel Dekker, 1993:201–54.
4. Schuppan D, Atkinson J, Ruehl M, Riecken EO. Alcohol and liver fibrosis – pathobiochemistry and treatment. Z Gastroenterol. 1995;33:546–50.
5. McClain C, Hill D, Schmidt J, Diehl AM. Cytokines and alcoholic liver disease. Sem Liver Dis. 1993;13:170–81.
6. Adachi Y, Bradford BA, Bojes HK, Thurman RG. Inactivation of Kupffer cells prevents early alcohol-induced liver injury. Hepatology. 1994;20:453–60.
7. Ramadori G. The stellate cell (Ito-cell, fat-storing cell, lipocyte, perisinusoidal cell) of the liver. New insights into pathophysiology of an intriguing cell. Virchows Arch B. 1991;61:147–58.
8. Floege J, Eng E, Young BA, Johnson RJ. Factors involved in the regulation of mesangial cell proliferation *in vitro* and *in vivo*. Kidney Intern. 1993;43 (S39): S47–54.
9. Elias J, Freundlich B, Kern JA, Rosenbloom J. Cytokine networks in the regulation of inflammation and fibrosis in the lung. Chest. 1990;97:1439–45.
10. Ross R. The pathogenesis of atherosclerosis: A perspective for the 1990s. Nature. 1993;362:801–9.
11. Schuppan D, Somasundaram R, Dieterich W, Ehnis T, Bauer M. The extracellular matrix in cellular differentiation and proliferation. In: Molecular and cell biological aspects of gastroenteropancreatic neuroendocrine tumour disease. Ann NY Acad Sci. 1994;733:87–102.

12. Schuppan D. Structure of the extracellular matrix in normal and fibrotic liver: Collagens and glycoproteins. Sem Liv Dis. 1990;10:1–10.
13. Schuppan D. Connective tissue polypeptides in serum as parameters to monitor antifibrotic treatment in hepatic fibrogenesis. J Hepatol. 1991;13 (Suppl 3):S17–25.
14. Schuppan D, Stölzel U, Oesterling C, Somasundaram R. Serum assays for liver fibrosis. J Hepatol 1995;22 (Suppl 2):82–8.
15. Arthur MJP. Matrix degradation in the liver. In: Surrenti C, Casini A, Milani S, Pinzani M, editors. Fat-storing cells and liver fibrosis. London: Kluwer, 1993:110–27.
16. Stetler-Stevenson WG, Liotta L, Kleiner DE. Role of matrix metalloproteinases in tumor invasion and metastasis. FASEB J. 1993;7:1434–41.
17. Nathan C, Sporn M. Cytokines in context. J Cell Biol. 1991;113:981–6.
18. Ruoslahti E, Yamaguchi Y. Proteoglycans as modulators of growth factor activities. Cell. 1991;64:867–9.
19. Rosenbloom J, Feldman G, Freundlich G, Jimenez SA. Transcriptional control of human diploid fibroblast collagen synthesis by interferon. Biochem Biophys Res Commun. 1984;123:365–72.
20. Castilla A, Prieto J, Fausto N. Transforming growth factors beta-1 and alfa in chronic liver disease: Effects of interferon-alfa therapy. N Engl J Med. 1991;324:933–40.
21. Manabe N, Chevallier M, Chossegros P *et al.* Interferon-α2b therapy reduces liver fibrosis in chronic non-A non-B hepatitis: A quantitative histologic evaluation. J Hepatol. 1993;18:1344–9.
22. Rockey DC, Maher JJ, Jarnagin WR, Gabbiani G, Friedman SL. Inhibition of rat lipocyte activation in culture by interferon-γ. Hepatology. 1992;16:776–84.
23. Ruwart MJ, Wilkinson KF, Rush BD *et al.* The integrated value of serum procollagen III peptide over time predicts hepatic hydroxyproline content and stainable collagen in a model of dietary cirrhosis in the rat. Hepatology. 1989;10:801–6.
24. Beno DWA, Espinal R, Edelstein BM, Davis BH. Administration of prostaglandin E1 analog reduces rat hepatic and Ito cell collagen gene expression and accumulation after bile duct ligation injury. Hepatology. 1993;17:707–14.
25. Unemori EN, Bauer EA, Amento EP. Relaxin alone and in conjunction with interferon-γ decreases collagen synthesis by cultured human scleroderma fibroblasts. J Invest Dermatol. 1992;99:337–42.
26. Lieber CS, Robins SJ, Li J *et al.* Phosphatidylcholine protects against fibrosis and cirrhosis in the baboon. Gastroenterology. 1994;106:152–9.
27. Li J, Kim CI, Leo MA, Mak KM, Rojkind M, Lieber CS. Polyunsaturated lecithin prevents acetaldehyde-mediated hepatic collagen accumulation by stimulating collagenase activity in cultured lipocytes. Hepatology. 1992;15:373–81.
28. Boigk G, Stroeter L, Waldschmidt J, Herbst H, Riecken EO, Schuppan D. Silymarin retards collagen accumulation in rat secondary biliary fibrosis. J Hepatol. 1995;23 (Suppl 1):142 (abstract).
29. Poo JI, Feldmann J, Erlinger S *et al.* Ursodeoxycholic acid limits liver histologic alterations and portal hypertension induced by bile duct ligation in the rat. Gastroenterology. 1992;102:1752–9.
30. Oesterling C, Aksü T, Somasundaram R *et al.* Serum markers of collagen synthesis and breakdown suggest an antifibrotic effect of ursodeoxycholic acid in patients with PBC stage I-IV. Gut. 1995;37 (Suppl 2):A121 (abstract).
31. Schuppan D. Vitamin A and liver fibrosis: Cure or villain. J Lab Clin Med. 1992;119:590–1.
32. Boigk G, Raetsch C, Stroeter L *et al.* Antifibrotic effect of pentoxifyllin in rat biliary fibrosis due to bile duct obstraction. J Hepatol. 1995;23 (Suppl 1):142 (abstract).
33. Hanauske-Abel HM. Prolyl 4-hydroxylase, a target enzyme for drug development. Design of suppressive agents and the *in vivo* effects of inhibitors and proinhibitors. J Hepatol. 1991;13 (Suppl3):S8–16.
34. Border WA, Ruoslahti E. Transforming growth factor-β in disease: The dark side of tissue repair. J Clin Invest. 1992;90:1–7.
35. Border WA, Noble NA, Yamamoto T *et al.* Natural inhibitor of transforming growth factor-β protects against scarring in experimental kidney disease. Nature. 1992;360:361–5.
36. Pinzani M, Gesualdo L, Sabbah GM, Abboud HE. Effects of platelet-derived growth factor and other mitogens on DNA synthesis and growth of cultured rat liver fat storing cells. J Clin Invest. 1989;84:1786–94.

37. Somasundaram R, Riecken EO, Schuppan D. Matrix-binding of platelet-derived growth factor (PDGF) in hepatic fibrosis is mediated by collagens type I, III, IV, V and VI. Gastroenterology. 1993;104:A998 (abstract).
38. Grinnell F. Fibroblasts, myofibroblasts and wound contraction. J Cell Biol. 1994;124:401–4.
39. Lin YC, Grinnell F. Decreased level of PDGF-stimulated receptor autophosphorylation by fibroblasts in mechanically relaxed collagen matrices. J Cell Biol. 1993;122:663–72.
40. Koivunen E, Ruoslahti E. Selection of peptides binding to the $\alpha 5\beta 1$ integrin from phage display library. J Biol Chem. 1993;268:20205–10.
41. Pfaff M, Tangemenn K, Müller B *et al.* Selective recognition of cyclic RGD peptides of NMR defined conformation by αIIbβ3, αVβ3, and $\alpha 5\beta 1$ integrins. J Biol Chem. 1994;269:20233–8.
42. Greenspoon N, Hershkoviz R, Alon R *et al.* Structural analysis of integrin recognition and the inhibition of integrin-mediated cell functions by novel nonpeptidic surrogates of the Arg-Gly-Asp sequence. Biochemistry. 1993;32:1001–8.
43. Tsukamoto H, Matsuoka M, French SW. Experimental models of hepatic fibrosis: An overview. Sem Liver Dis. 1990;10:56–65.
44. Perez Tamayo R. Is cirrhosis of the liver experimentally produced by CCl_4 an adequate model of human cirrhosis? Hepatology. 1984;3:112–20.
45. Zimmermann T, Gardemann A, Machnik G, Dargel R, Jungermann K. Metabolic and hemodynamic responses of bivascularly perfused rat liver to nerve stimulation, noradrenaline, acetylcholine and glucagon in thioacetamide-induced liver cirrhosis. Hepatology. 1992;15:464–70.
46. Kontouras J, Billing BH, Scheuer PJ. Prolonged bile duct obstruction: A new experimental model for cirrhosis in the rat. Br J Exp Pathol. 1984;65:305–11.
47. Abdi W, Millan JC, Mezey E. Sampling variability on percutaneous liver biopsy. Arch Int Med. 1979;139:667–9.
48. Risteli L, Risteli J. Noninvasive methods for detection of of organ fibrosis. In: Rojkind M, editor. Focus on connective tissue in health and disease. Boca Raton: CRC Press, 1990:61–98.
49. Plebani M, Burlina A. Biochemical markers of hepatic fibrosis. Clin Biochem. 1991;24:219–39.
50. Guseva NG, Anikina NV, Myllylä R, Risteli J, Risteli J. Markers of collagen and basement membrane metabolism in sera of patients with progressive systemic sclerosis. Ann Rheum Dis. 1991;50:481–6.
51. Eberhardt K, Jensen LT, Hørslev-Petersen K, Pettersson H, Lorenzen I, Wollheim F. Serum aminoterminal type III procollagen peptide in early rheumatoid arthritis: Relation to disease activity and progression of joint damage. Clin Exp Rheumatol. 1990;8:335–40.
52. Hartman DJ, Laurent PA, Jacob BA, Lafuma C. Serum and urinary markers for lung elastin and collagen degradation. In: Hirsch A, Goldberg M, Martin JP, Masse R, editors. Prevention of respiratory diseases. New York: Marcel Dekker, 1993:345–72.
53. Haukkipuro K, Melkko J, Risteli L, Kairoluoma MI, Risteli J. Connective tissue response to major surgery and postoperative infection. Eur J Clin Invest. 1992;22:333–40.
54. Keller F, Rehbein C, Schwarz A *et al.* Increased procollagen III production in patients with kidney diseases. Nephron. 1988;50:332–7.
55. Keller F, Ser YL, Schuppan D. Raised concentrations of the carboxyterminal propeptide of type IV (basement membrane) procollagen (NC1) in serum and urine of patients with glomerulonephritis. Eur J Clin Invest. 1992;22:175–81.
56. Marder K, Keller F, Schuppan D. Circulating type VI collagen and undulin in patients with kidney diseases, after kidney transplantation and on hemodialysis. Clin Nephrol. 1995;44:178–84.
57. Risteli L, Risteli J, Tomas C, Zhu GG, Kauppila A. Aminoterminal propeptide of type III procollagen in ovarian cancer. Acta Obstet Gynecol Scand. 1992;155:S99–103.
58. Risteli L, Risteli J. Biochemical markers of bone metabolism. Ann Med. 1993;25:385–93.
59. Trinchet JC, Hartman DJ, Pateron D *et al.* Serum type I collagen and N-terminal peptide of type III procollagen in chronic hepatitis. Relationship to liver histology and conventional liver tests. J Hepatol. 1991;12:139–44.
60. Shahin M, Schuppan D, Waldherr R *et al.* Serum procollagen peptides and collagen type VI for the assessment of activity and degree of hepatic fibrosis in schistosomiasis and alcoholic liver disease. Hepatology. 1992;15:637–44.
61. Niemelä O, Risteli L, Sotaniemi EA, Risteli J. Type IV collagen and laminin-related antigens in human sera in alcoholic liver disease. Eur J Clin Invest. 1985;15:132–7.

62. Kropf J, Gressner AM, Negwer A. Efficacy of serum laminin measurement for diagnosis of fibrotic liver diseases. Clin Chem. 1988;34:2026–30.
63. Schuppan D, Besser M, Schwarting R, Hahn EG. Radioimmunoassay for the carboxyterminal crosslinking domain of type IV (basement membrane) procollagen in body fluids. J Clin Invest. 1986;78:241–8.
64. Hayasaka A, Schuppan D, Ohnishi K, Okuda K, Hahn EG. Serum concentrations of the carboxyterminal cross-linking domain of procollagen type IV (NC1) and the aminoterminal propeptide of procollagen type III (PIIIP) in chronic liver disease. J Hepatol. 1991;10:17–22.
65. Yamada S, Suou T, Kawasaki H, Yoshikawa N. Clinical significance of serum 7S collagen in various liver diseases. Clin Biochem. 1992;25:467–70.
66. Yabu K, Kiyosawa K, Mori H, Matsumoto A, Yoshizawa K, Tanaka E. Serum collagen type IV for the assessment of fibrosis and resistance to interferon therapy in chronic hepatitis C. Scand J Gastroenterol. 1994;29:474–9.
67. Hiramatsu N, Hayashi N, Kasahara A *et al.* Improvement of liver fibrosis in chronic hepatitis C patients treated with interferon alpha. J Hepatol. 1995;22:135–42.
68. Murawaki Y, Ikuta Y, Nishimura Y, Koda M, Kawasaki H. Serum markers for connective tissue turnover in patients with chronic hepatitis B and chronic hepatitis C: A comparative analysis. J Hepatol. 1995;23:145–52.
69. Raedsch R, Stiehl A, Sieg A, Walther S, Kommerell B. Biliary excretion of procollagen type III peptide in healthy humans and in patients with cirrhosis of the liver. Gastroenterology. 1983;85:1265–70.
70. Laurent TC, Fraser RE. Hyaluronan. FASEB J. 1992;6:2397–404.
71. Erikson S, Fraser JRE, Laurent TC, Pertoft K, Smedsrød B. Endothelial cells are a site of uptake and degradation of hyaluronic acid in the liver. Exp Cell Res. 1983;144:223–8.
72. Smedsrød B. Aminoterminal propeptide of type III procollagen is cleared from the circulation by receptor mediated endocytosis in liver endothelial cells. Collagen Relat Res. 1988;8:3.75–88.
73. Smedsrød B, Melkko J, Risteli L, Risteli J. Circulating carboxyterminal propeptide of type I procollagen is cleared mainly via the mannose receptor of liver endothelial cells. Biochem J. 1990;271:345–50.
74. Smedsrød B, Paulsson M, Johansson S. Uptake and degradation *in vivo* and *in vitro* of laminin and nitrogen by rat liver cells. Biochem J. 1989;261:37–42.
75. Thorbjørn Jensen L, Henriksen JH, Risteli J, Olesen HP, Nielsen MD, Lorenzen, I. Fate of circulating aminoterminal propeptide of type III procollagen in conscious pigs. Am J Physiol. 1993;265:R139–145.
76. Schuppan D, Kim KY, Teike T, Hahn EG, Riecken EO. Alteration of the metabolism of circulating procollagen IV propeptide (NC1), but not of procollagen III propeptide (PIIIP) in biliary fibrosis. Gastroenterology. 1989;96:A658(abstract).
77. Hayasaka A Koch J, Schuppan D, Maddrey WC, Hahn EG. The serum concentrations of the aminoterminal propeptide of procollagen type III and the hepatic content of mRNA for the $\alpha 1$ chain of procollagen type III in carbon tetrachloride-induced rat liver fibrogenesis. J Hepatol. 1991;13:328–38.
78. Torres-Salinas M, Pares A, Caballeria J, *et al.* Serum procollagen type III peptide as a marker of hepatic fibrogenesis in alcoholic hepatitis. Gastroenterology. 1986;90:1241–6.
79. Rohde H, Vargas L, Hahn E, Kalbfleisch H, Bruguera M, Timpl R. Radioimmunoassay for type III procollagen peptide and its application to human liver disease. Eur J Clin Invest. 1979;9:451–9.
80. Weigand K, Zaugg PY, Frei A, Zimmermann A. Long-term follow-up of serum N-terminal propeptide of collagen type III levels in patients with chronic liver diseases. Hepatology. 1984;4:835–8.
81. Annoni G, Cargnel A, Colombo M, Hahn EG. Persistant elevation of the aminoterminal peptide of procollagen type III in serum of patients with acute viral hepatitis distinguishes chronic active hepatitis from resolving or chronic persistent hepatitis. J Hepatol. 1986;2:379–88.
82. Bentsen Ko, Hørslev-Petersen K, Junker P, et al. Serum aminoterminal procollagen type III peptide in acute viral hepatitis. A long-term follow-up study. J Hepatol. 1986;2:370–8.
83. Ballardini G, Faccani A, Bianchi FB *et al.* Steroid treatment lowers hepatic fibroplasia, as explored by serum aminoterminal procollagen III peptide, in chronic liver disease. Liver. 1984;4:348–52.
84. McCullough AJ, Stassen WN, Wiesner RH, Czaja AJ. Serum type III procollagen peptide concentrations in serum in severe chronic active hepatitis; Relationship to cirrhosis and disease activity. Hepatology. 1987;7:49–54.

85. Eriksson S, Zettervall O. The N-terminal propeptide of collagen type III in serum as a prognostic indicator in primary biliary cirrhosis. J Hepatol. 1986;2:370–8.
86. Babbs C, Hunt LP, Haboubi NY, Smith A, Rowan BP, Warnes TW. Type III procollagen peptide; A marker of disease activity and prognosis in primary biliary cirrhosis. Lancet. 1988;1:1021–4.
87. Beukers A, van Zanten RAA, Schalm SW. Serial determination of type III procollagen amino propeptide serum levels in patients with histologically progressive and non-progressive primary biliary cirrhosis. J Hepatol. 1992;14:22–9.
88. Rohde H, Langer I, Krieg T, Timpl R. Serum and urine analysis of the aminoterminal procollagen peptide type III by radioimmunoassay with antibody Fab fragments. Collagen Rel Res. 1983;3:371–9.
89. Risteli J, Niemi S, Trivedi P, Mäentausta O, Mowat AP, Risteli L. Rapid equilibrium assay for the amino-terminal propeptide of human type III procollagen. Clin Chem. 1988;34:715–8.
90. Teran JC, Mullen KD, Hoofnagle JH, McCullough AJ. Decrease in serum levels of markers of hepatic connective tissue turnover during and after treatment of chronic hepatitis B with alfa interferon. Hepatology. 1994;19:849–56.
91. Capra F, Casaril M, Gabrielli GB, *et al.* α-Interferon in the treatment of chronic viral hepatitis; Effects on fibrogenesis serum markers. J Hepatol. 1993;18:112–8.
92. Camps J, Castilla A, Ruiz J, Civeira MP, Prieto J. Randomised trial of lymphoblastoid α-interferon in chronic hepatitis C. Effects on inflammation, fibrogenesis and viremia. J Hepatol. 1993;17:390–6.
93. Gallorini A, Plebani M, Pontisso P, Chemello L, Mantovani G, Alberti A. Serum markers of hepatic fibrogenesis in chronic hepatitis C treated with alfa-2A interferon. J Hepatol. 1994;14:257–64.
94. Suou T, Hosho K, Kishimoto Y, Horie Y, Kawasaki H. Long-term decrease in serum N-terminal propeptide of type III procollagen in patients with chronic hepatitis C treated with interferon alfa. Hepatology. 1995;22:426–31.
95. Schvarcz R, Glaumann H, Weiland O, Norkrans G, Wejstal R, Fryden A. Histological outcome in interferon alpha-2b treated patients with chronic posttransfusion non-A, non-B hepatitis. Liver. 1991;11:30–8.
96. Schuppan D, Rühlmann T, Hahn EG. Radioimmunoassay for human type VI collagen and its application to tissue and body fluids. Anal Biochem. 1985;148:238–47.
97. Trivedi P, Cheeseman P, Portman B, Mowat AP. Serum type III procollagen peptide as a non-invasive marker of liver damage during infancy and childhood in extrahepatic biliary atresia, idiopathic hepatitis of infancy and $\alpha 1$ antitrypsin deficiency. Clin Chim Acta. 1986; 161:137–46.
98. Danne T, Decker J, Schuppan D *et al.* Serum levels of laminin P1 and of type IV collagen in healthy children and in children with insulin-dependent diabetes mellitus. In: Gubler MC, Sternberg M, editors. Progress in basement membrane research. Renal and related aspects in health and disease. London: John Libbey Eurotext, 1988: 315–22.
99. Gerling B, Schuppan D, Hanisch U, Luck W, Becker M. Split products of extracellular matrix proteins: Relevance in diagnosis and follow-up of pediatric liver fibrosis. Gut. 1995;37 (Suppl 2):A122 (abstract).
100. Schuppan D, Cantaluppi C, Becker J *et al.* Undulin, an extracellular matrix glycoprotein associated with collagen fibrils. J Biol Chem. 1990;264:8823–32.
101. Shahin M, Schuppan D, Waldhern R *et al.* Circulating enzyme activities of collagen turnover and undulin in patients with various degrees of schistosomiasis and alcoholic liver cirrhosis. Hepato-Gastroenterology. 1995;42:22–6.
102. Stickel F, Schuppan D, Oesterling C *et al.* Serum undulin as an indicator of early alterations of hepatic connective tissue turnover due to alcohol. Alcohol Alcoholism. 1995;30:4 (abstract).
103. Nyberg A, Lindquist U, Engström-Laurent A. Serum hyaluronan and aminoterminal propeptide type III procollagen in primary biliary cirrhosis: Relation to clinical symptoms, liver histopathology and outcome. J Int Med. 1992;231:485–91.
104. Guechot J, Poupon RE, Giral P, Balkau B, Giboudeau J, Poupon R. Relationship between procollagen III aminoterminal propeptide and hyaluronan serum levels and histological fibrosis in primary biliary cirrhosis and chronic viral hepatitis C. J Hepatol. 1994;20:388–93.
105. Guechot J, Loria A, Serfaty L, Giral P, Giboudeau J, Poupon R. Serum hyaluronan as a marker of liver cirrosis in chronic viral hepatitis C: Effect of α-interferon therapy. J Hepatol. 1995;22:22–6.

106. Ramadori G, Zöhrens G, Manns M *et al.* Serum hyaluronate and type III procollagen aminoterminal propeptide concentration in chronic liver disease. Relationship to cirrhosis and disease activity. Eur J Clin Invest. 1991;21:323–30.
107. Pares A, Deulofeu R, Gimenez A *et al.* Serum hyaluronate reflects liver inflammation and fibrogenesis in alcoholic liver disease. J Hepatol. 1995;23 (Suppl 3):139.
108. Yamauchi M, Nakajima H, Ohata M *et al.* Detection of fibronectin receptor in sera: Its clinical significance as a parameter of hepatic fibrosis. Hepatology. 1991;14:244–50.
109. Hynes RO. Integrins: Versatility, modulation and signaling in cell adhesion. Cell 1992;69:11–25.
110. Van Eyken P, Sciot R, Desmet VJ. Expression of the novel extracellular matrix component tenascin in normal and diseased human liver. J Hepatol. 1990;11:43–52.
111. Yamauchi M, Mizuhara Y, Maezawa Y, Ida G. Serum tenascin levels in chronic liver disease. Liver. 1994;14:148–53.
112. Libuda P, Oesterling C, Aksü T *et al.* Tenascin is a serum parameter of lobular but not portal fibrogenesis in chronic liver diseases. Hepatology. 1995;22:369A(abstr.).
113. Maruyama X, Feinman L, Fainsilber Z, Nakano M, Okazaki I, Lieber CS. Mammalian collagenase increases in early alcoholic liver disease and decreases with cirrhosis. Life Sci. 1982;30:1379–84.
114. Milani S, Herbst H, Schuppan D *et al.* Differential expression of matrix-metalloproteinase-1 and -2 genes in normal and fibrotic human liver. Am J Pathol. 1994;144:528–37.
115. Murawaki Y, Koda M, Yamada S, Kawasaki H, Shima H, Burkhardt H. Serum collagenase activity in patients with chronic liver disease. J Hepatol. 1993;18:328–34.
116. Herbst H, Wege T, Bechstein OW, Neuhaus P, Gressner AM, Schuppan D. Expression of TIMP-1 and -2 in normal and fibrotic liver. J Hepatol. 1995;23 (Suppl 1):140 (abstract).
117. Li JJ, Rosman AS, Leo MA, Nagai Y, Lieber CS. Tissue inhibitor of metalloproteinase is increased in the serum of precirrhotic and cirrhotic alcoholic patients and can serve as a marker of fibrosis. Hepatology. 1994;19:1418–23.

13
Surrogate markers to assess efficiency of treatment in chronic liver diseases: new biochemical indices

G. RAMADORI and F. POLZIEN

In chronic liver diseases surrogate markers are used to differentiate hepatocyte necrosis and cholestasis, as well as fibrogenesis and cirrhosis with increased connective tissue deposition and remodelling of hepatic structure. The decrease of functional hepatic tissue can also be estimated by biochemical markers. Other markers are available for estimating severity of inflammation, portal hypertension and porto–systemic shunting and indicators for metabolic and clearance capacity have been described. Furthermore there may be surrogate markers for several specific hepatic functions. In this chapter we will discuss surrogate markers for hepatocyte necrosis, cholestasis, cirrhosis, inflammation and metabolic clearance capacity. In particular we will focus on biochemical indices as surrogate markers other than those which are considered to be classic (i.e. serum transaminases, alkaline phosphatase, bilirubin, etc.).

SOLUBLE INTERCELLULAR ADHESION MOLECULE TYPE 1 (sICAM-1) AS INDICATOR OF HEPATOCELLULAR NECROSIS

This adhesion molecule is a member of the immunoglobulin superfamily. The molecule contains multiple immunoglobulin like-domains and it can become expressed on the plasma membrane of a great number of different cells (lympohcytes, hepatocytes, biliary epithelial cells, endothelial cells). Activated leukocytes can show an increased production of ICAM-1.

The natural ligand is the CD11a/18, the so-called leukocyte function associated antigen-1 (LFA-1). ICAM-1 mediates the adhesion of T-lymphocytes to B cells, macrophages, endothelial cells and other target cells (e.g. hepatocytes, biliary epithelial cells). ICAM-1 gene expression can be induced or increased in different cell populations, and also in hepatocytes. The expression of ICAM-1 in some cells can be induced by proinflammatory cytokines. Also the action of viral proteins, as has been demonstrated by the X-protein of the hepatitis B virus, can induce ICAM-1 expression[1,2].

ICAM-1 is released from cells to the extracellular compartment and a soluble ICAM-1 form can be found in serum.

In 1992, Adams *et al.* measured the concentration of ICAM-1 in the serum of patients with different chronic liver diseases[3]. In patients with primary biliary cirrhosis, primary sclerosing cholangitis, alcoholic cirrhosis, cryptogenic cirrhosis or hepatitis B, markedly elevated concentrations of circulating ICAM-1 were found compared to healthy controls. Highest sICAM-1 serum concentrations were found in patients with cholestatic liver disease – primary biliary cirrhosis and primary sclerosing cholangitis – compared to other chronic liver diseases. Activated lymphocytes were speculated as a possible source of circulating ICAM-1. Furthermore, circulating ICAM-1 could even play a potential immunoregulatory role, underlining the immunopathogenesis of these cholestatic liver diseases.

Recently we found increased sICAM-1 concentrations in patients with acute and chronic hepatitis, drug-induced hepatitis and active cirrhosis[4]. Twenty patients with acute viral hepatitis, 6 patients with drug-induced acute hepatitis, 17 with chronic persistent cirrhosis, 42 with chronic active cirrhosis and 25 with active cirrhosis were studied. Serum concentration of ICAM-1 was significantly increased in patients with acute hepatitis, chronic active hepatitis or active cirrhosis[4].

The serum level was dependent on the degree of inflammatory activity and there was a significant correlation between the level of transaminases and serum concentration of ICAM-1. The ICAM-1 serum concentration decreased in patients with autoimmune liver disease, when remission was reached under immunosuppressive therapy. This was true for both patients with chronic active hepatitis and patients with an active cirrhosis. The ICAM-1 serum levels in patients with acute viral or drug-induced hepatitis were comparable or even higher than those measured in serum of patients with chronic active hepatitis or active cirrhosis. We also could find no difference between serum levels of ICAM-1 in patients with autoimmune hepatitis and patients with viral-induced chronic hepatitis, when patients with a comparable inflammatory degree of liver disease were compared[4]. These studies indicate that serum ICAM-1 in acute and chronic liver disease is probably released from necrotic hepatocytes instead of from activated immunocells, and could therefore be a marker for hepatocellular damage (Table 1).

Table 1 Surrogate markers for hepatocyte necrosis

AST
ALT
AST/ALT >2
(Alcoholic liver damage)
Coagulation proteins
(Factor V)
ICAM-1

SOLUBLE INTERCELLULAR ADHESION MOLECULE TYPE 1 (sICAM-1) AS A POSSIBLE INDICATOR OF CHOLESTASIS

The diagnostic value of ICAM-1 in cholestatic diseases will be discussed. The possible cause of increased serum ICAM-1 in cholestatic liver disease can be due to increased synthesis by biliary cells as well as by inflammatory cells. However, decreased elimination through the bile could also result in an increased serum level of ICAM-1. We studied the concentration of sICAM-1 in the serum of patients with intrahepatic, and also extrahepatic cholestasis. We measured the concentration of ICAM-1 in patients with primary biliary cirrhosis, before and during treatment with ursodeoxycholic acid and we also measured the concentration of soluble ICAM-1 in the bile[5].

sICAM-1 concentration was elevated in patients with primary biliary cirrhosis (PBC) and the increase was highest in patients with PBC stage 4. In PBC stages (1 and 2), the ICAM-1 serum concentration was a better marker for cholestasis than alkaline phospatase. Furthermore, in PBC, the early histological stages (1 and 2) could be differentiated with high specificity (0.85) and sensitivity (0.95) from late-stage PBC (stages 3 and 4)[5].

In patients in which ursodeoxycholic acid was effective in inducing a decrease in cholestasis markers, ICAM-1 serum concentration also decreased. Interestingly, sICAM-1 serum concentration was increased, not only in patients with intrahepatic cholestasis, but also in patients with extrahepatic cholestasis with no signs of inflammation. In some bile samples, we found measurable levels of ICAM-1 and the concentration was even as high as the concentration in the serum.

Our data suggest that soluble ICAM-1 may be eliminated through the bile, and that intra-, as well as extrahepatic cholestasis may induce an increase in serum concentration. These data are partly in agreement with those recently published[6]. ICAM-1 serum concentrations were elevated in PBC patients and levels were highest in patients with stage 3 and 4 disease. The serum level of IL-2 receptor was also elevated and it was concluded that both markers could be an indication for the immunohepatogenesis of the disease. Our data show, at least in part, a decreased elimination of those proteins which could be responsible for the increased serum levels in cholestasis.

Recently, it was found that expression of ICAM-1 on liver cells was only increased in stage 3 of primary sclerosing cholangitis, but in PBC there was no significant expression of ICAM-1 in correlation with histological stage 3 and 4 or in extent of inflammation[7]. We and other authors also found that the serum level was increased most in late-stage disease and the inflammation is histologically insignificant.

Soluble ICAM-1 appears to be a new marker, at least for intrahepatic cholestasis (Table 2), and can differentiate between early- and late-stage PBC with high specificity and sensitivity.

Table 2 Surrogate markers for cholestasis

Alkaline phosphatase
γ-GT, bilirubin
ICAM-1

SURROGATE MARKERS FOR LIVER FUNCTION

Non macrophage-dependent clearance function

It is known that hyaluronic acid (HA) circulating in the blood is rapidly taken up by the liver; therefore, metabolism of HA can serve as an indicator of reduced clearance capacity of the liver tissue and may have important diagnostic use in patients with liver disease (i.e. cirrhosis).

Hyaluronan or hyaluronic acid is an unbranched, high molecular weight polysaccharide, which is widely distributed in extracellular space. The highest concentration is found in the lymph; only a small portion is found in the blood and this portion is cleared by the sinusoidal endothelial cells of the liver. The half-life of circulating hyaluronic acid is 2.5 to 5 minutes. Several years ago, a method to measure hyaluronan concentration in the serum was established by Swedish scientists and we used this method to measure the concentration of serum hyaluronan in patients with acute or chronic liver diseases[8].

Hyaluronan serum concentration was significantly increased in patients with acute hepatitis, as well as in patients with active cirrhosis. In patients with autoimmune chronic liver diseases, hyaluronan serum concentration was studied before and during immunosupression. While the hyaluronan serum concentration in patients with chronic active hepatitis, was not significantly different to that in controls at the time of remission, it remained elevated in patients with inactive cirrhosis. This indicates that hyaluronan is increased in acute as well as in chronic liver disease where tissue necrosis occurs; it is also increased in patients with inactive cirrhosis, where elimination of hyaluronic acid by endothelial cells may be reduced because of reduced numbers of endothelial cells and also because of shunting of the portal blood (Table 3).

Table 3 Surrogate markers as indicators of reduced clearance capacity of the liver (e.g. cirrhosis)

Hyaluronic acid
MEGX formation

It may be interesting to mention some results obtained by measuring the concentration of hyaluronic acid in the serum of patients with chronic hepatitis B infection before and after interferon-α therapy[8]. Hyaluronan serum concentration was increased in these patients, and the concentration was further increased by interferon-α. In both responders and non-responders, the increase induced by interferon-α was also found in patients with low inflammatory activity, such as in chronic persistent hepatitis, but was not found in normal volunteers. This could indicate that interferon-α either induced an increase in hyaluronan release or a decrease in elimination through the endothelial cells. Interestingly, the measurement of hyaluronic acid could be a surrogate marker for compliance in patients with chronic liver diseases under treatment with interferon-α[9].

Lidocaine metabolism and MEGX formation as markers of liver function and/or liver circulation

A new method for assessment of hepatic function was evaluated a few years ago. It is known that lidocaine is mainly metabolized with a high first-pass effect at the cytochrome P450 complex in hepatocytes. By application of lidocaine intravenously (1 mg/kg body weight), the kinetics of its deacetylation at the liver cytochrome P450 complex can be measured within minutes.

Monoethylglycinexylidide (MEGX) is a stable product and serves as an indicator for the metabolizing capacity of the liver. In patients with liver disease, especially in patients with cirrhotic livers, the metabolizing capacity of the functional liver tissue is also dependent on porto–systemic shunt flow. Therefore MEGX formation can be used for quantitative assessment of functional liver tissue and portal–shunt flow[10] (Table 3).

In a patient with HCV induced active cirrhosis and two previous episodes of oesophageal variceal bleeding, routine laboratory values (AST/ALT) were evaluated before starting interferon therapy. MEGX production was initially reduced. During interferon therapy there was a complete biochemical normalization and MEGX formation was within the normal range. There were also no episodes of bleeding. This may indicate that in some way the suppression of inflammatory activity in the liver induces an increase in MEGX production. This could be due to the improvement of liver circulation and/or to an increase of hepatic functional mass by reduced damage.

In recent years a great number of cytokines, cytokine receptors and several other substances have been measured in the serum of patients with liver diseases. None appears to be a suitable candidate for monitoring patients with chronic liver disease.

References

1. Hue K-Q, Yu CH, Vierling JM. Up-regulation of intercellular adhesion molecule 1 transcription by hepatitis B virus X protein. Proc Natl Acad Sci USA. 1992;89:11441–5.
2. Mihm S, Ramadori G. HBX-induzierte ICAM-1 Expression. Z Gastroenterol. 1994;32:126–8.
3. Adams DH, Mainolfi E, Burra P *et al.* Detection of circulating intercellular adhesion molecule-1 in chronic liver diseases. Hepatology. 1992;16:810–4.
4. Zöhrens G, Armbrust T, Pirzer U, Meyer zum Büschenfelde KH, Ramadori G. Intercellular adhesion molecule-1 concentration in sera of patients with acute and chronic liver disease: Relationship to disease activity and cirrhosis. Hepatology. 1993;18:798–802.
5. Polzien F, Hilgers RA, Ramadori G. Increased intercellular adhesion molecule-1 serum concentration in cholestasis. J Hepatol. 1996 (in press).
6. Lim AG, Jazrawi RP, Ahmed HA *et al.* Soluble intercellular adhesion molecule-1 in primary biliary cirrhosis: Relationship with disease stage, immune activity and cholestasis. Hepatology. 1994;20:882–8.
7. Bloom S, Fleming K, Chapman R. Adhesion molecule expression in primary sclerosing chlangitis and primary biliary cirrhosis. Gut. 1995;36:604–9.
8. Ramadori G, Zöhrens G, Manns M *et al.* Serum hyaluronate and type III procollagen aminoterminal propeptide concentration in chronic liver disease. Relationship to cirrhosis and disease activity. Eur J Clin Invest. 1991;21:323–30.
9. Zöhrens G, Armbrust T, Meyer zum Büschenfelde KH, Ramadori G. Interferon-α2a increases serum concentration of hyaluronic acid and type III procollagen aminoterminal propeptide in patients with chronic hepatitis B virus infection. Digest Dis Sci. 1994;39:2007–13.
10. Oellerich M, Burdelski M, Lautz HU, Schulz M, Schmidt FW, Herrmann H. Lidocaine metabolite formation as a measure of liver function in patients with cirrhosis. Ther Drug Monitor. 1990;12:219–26.

14
Liver biopsy as a surrogate marker in chronic liver disease

B. PORTMANN

INTRODUCTION

Although liver biopsy has been somewhat dislodged from its previously undisputed role of 'gold standard' in the diagnosis of chronic liver disease, needle biopsies remain an important tool both to secure the initial diagnosis and to evaluate degree of activity, stage and progression of the liver lesion. Many therapeutic trials have used, and are still using, histology to evaluate potential benefits of various individual drugs. Consequently, there is a need for reliable scoring systems that would be reproducible and allow comparison between different institutions.

The aim of this chapter is not to provide new scoring systems which would only add to the confusion following recent discussions on terminology and proposals for grading and staging of histological changes, but to review the ones currently used to evaluate histological activity and disease stage in chronic hepatitis and in chronic cholestatic liver disorders.

CHRONIC HEPATITIS

Nomenclature of chronic hepatitis

Recent editorials and review articles[1–4] have stressed the need to revise the histological classification of chronic hepatitis. The 25-year-old classification into chronic persistent (CPH), chronic active (CAH) and chronic lobular (CLH) hepatitis[5] has certainly passed the test of time and has been most useful to both pathologists and clinicians, but it no longer permits incorporation of the impressive progress which has been achieved in the understanding of chronic hepatitis, in particular the recognition of various aetiologies – viral hepatitis B, C and D – and the parallel progress which has been made in therapy and in the understanding of pathogenic mechanisms. In addition, the initial distinction between CPH and CAH became misinterpreted as representing separate disorders, rather than different grades of severity[4]. Over the past decade, longitudinal studies in chronic hepatitis have clearly shown that disease course, prognosis and response to treatment, depend as much on the aetiology, state of viral replication and host factors as they do on histological features at a given time in the evolution of the disease. In chronic hepatitis C for example, the histology is often that of a low-grade activity which would have been classified on the borderline between CPH and CAH in the old nomenclature; in spite of this, cirrhosis develops in a high proportion of cases suggesting that in this situation, piecemeal necrosis or interface hepatitis, the distinguishing feature of CPH and CAH, may be only one of several types of parenchymal damage in chronic hepatitis. Consequently, most proposals for a revised classification recommend a system which should be primarily based on aetiology, e.g. chronic hepatitis B, C, D[6,7], the term 'chronic' being considered superfluous for the autoimmune forms which are chronic by definition[8]. Within these categories, a histological grade of activity is indicated based on subjective grading of the necro-inflammatory process into minimal, mild, moderate or severe (see Table 1). The staging of the lesion is an attempt to position the lesion on an imaginary time line from onset of disease to cirrhosis. This is best achieved in grading fibrosis into mild (portal fibrous expansion), moderate (periportal radiating septa), severe (bridging septa) or cirrhosis. Thus examples of final diagnosis in this system are as follows: chronic hepatitis B, moderate activity with moderate fibrosis; chronic hepatitis C, mild activity with cirrhosis; autoimmune hepatitis, severe activity with severe fibrosis. Due to the lack of specificity of the histological features, aetiological diagnoses often require information on serological data which in most instances are available at the time of or shortly after the biopsy being performed. The grading of the necro-inflammatory activity is obtained by estimating overall the portal inflammation, interface hepatitis and intra-acinar inflammation and liver cell damage using accepted criteria. This is sufficient to establish the diagnosis, to institute a specific treatment or to enter the patient in a clinical trial of therapy, and, in the case of autoimmune hepatitis, to adjust the level or consider withdrawal of immunosuppression. In chronic viral hepatitis, particularly when

Table 1 Terminology of chronic hepatitis

New	*Old*	*Morphological*
Chronic hepatitis B, C, *or* **D,** *or* **autoimmune hepatitis**		
with **minimal**	**NSH**/CPH/**CLH**	Mild portal hepatitis
mild	**CPH**/CLH	Portal ± lobular hepatitis
	CAH mild	± mild PMN
moderate	**CAH** moderate	Periportal (interface) hepatitis (PMN)
or **severe activity**	**CAH** severe	Severe PMN ± bridging necrosis
with **no**		No fibrosis
mild		Portal fibrosis
moderate		Periportal radiating fibrous septa
or **severe fibrosis**		Bridging fibrous septa
or **cirrhosis**		Cirrhosis

Abbreviations: NSH, non-specific hepatitis; CPH, chronic persistent hepatitis; CAH, chronic active hepatitis; CLH, chronic lobular hepatitis; PMN, piecemeal necrosis baseline biopsies have to be compared with protocol specimens taken after treatment, and for other research endeavours, there is a need for precise scoring systems which can more readily be analysed.

Grading and staging of chronic hepatitis

Semi-quantitative grading and staging systems have been devised to allocate numerical scores to the histological features which are thought to indicate the severity and the progression of chronic hepatitis on an imaginary time line from onset of disease to cirrhosis[4]. They can supplement, but not replace, verbal descriptions in routine diagnostic practice. The following criteria should be met by a good scoring system and taken into account by pathologists and clinicians when selecting a method:

1. It should be appropriate for the intended project, but it may incorporate features which, though not of immediate interest, might emerge as important in the future; this raises the question of whether a single system should be applied to all aetiologies, considering for example, the usually low grade activity and absence of confluent parenchymal necrosis in chronic hepatitis C, which markedly contrast with the severe activity and frequent bridging necrosis observed in untreated autoimmune hepatitis.
2. The system should be simple and convenient to use by different observers, yet should provide sufficient information of potential clinical or scientific value.
3. It should be reproducible, i.e. associated with a low intra- and inter-observer variation when tested by the kappa statistic[9].
4. It should be clinically relevant, and ideally have a prognostic value, although validation in this respect might be difficult due to the lack of baseline studies on the natural history of untreated chronic hepatitis.

Several different scoring systems have been proposed[1,6,10–12]. By far the most widely used is the Histological Activity Index (HAI) of Knodell *et al.*[10] which has allowed a crude meta-analysis of results in many therapeutic trials of various forms of chronic hepatitis. This wide acceptance is certainly one of the many advantages of the system, but recently some shortcomings have been highlighted, suggesting a need for modification. In particular the grading scores of the necro-inflammatory activity (components 1, 2 and 3 of the HAI) should be clearly separated from the stage (component 4 of the HAI), which is a measure of fibrosis and architectural alteration, i.e. the structural progression of the disease, which is currently believed to be the consequence of the necro-inflammatory process. The first component could be subdivided to allow separate assessment of piecemeal (interface) and bridging necrosis which may have different prognostic implications[6,7,13]. In all four categories of the HAI, a range of scores from 0 to 10 or 0 to 4 is given, but some of the numbers are omitted and pathologists may be in doubt as to whether the omitted scores are permissible. A further factor to consider is that the scores of the HAI represent discontinuous variables of undetermined value, and must be treated as such in statistical evaluation.

Although widely used, the reproducibility of HAI scores has not been adequately tested. Recently it has been shown that inter-observer agreement was only fair for the major components 1, 2 and 3 of the Knodell system, acceptable degree of concordance of the global HAI being related mainly to the high degree of concordance of the fibrosis score[11]. Another comparative study has shown that inter-observer variation was less using the simplified Scheuer system[1] for the necro-inflammatory components, whereas similar results were obtained with either system for fibrosis[14]. The HAI scores, except for component 2 (intralobular degeneration and focal necrosis) were also shown to have no predictive value as to response to interferon therapy in chronic hepatitis C[15]. The above considerations raise the question of what scoring system should be used in the future. One approach has been to improve the HAI. It is universally accepted that grading and staging should be scored separately and there is also increasing agreement as to the types of necro-inflammation which should be scored separately, namely periportal or periseptal interface hepatitis (piecemeal necrosis), confluent necrosis, focal parenchymal necrosis and inflammation, and portal inflammation. These issues have been extensively discussed by Desmet *et al.*[6], and more recently in a special article by an International Group[16]. The latter article proposes a modification of the HAI system to take the above criticisms into account; the model is being tested and may well require further refinement. As demonstrated by French pathologists[11], more precise definitions, simplification of grading and prior agreement of criteria between all observers, are essential steps to improve reproducibility.

CHRONIC CHOLESTATIC LIVER DISEASE

Primary biliary cirrhosis

The stratification of *primary biliary cirrhosis* (PBC) into four histological stages has survived intact over the years, except for subtle changes in the designation of the stages, all systems agreeing with stage 4 being that of established cirrhosis[17–19]. Partly due to the uneven distribution of the changes within the liver as evidenced in livers removed at transplantation, there has frequently been a poor correlation between the clinical state of the patient and the apparent histological staging. Nevertheless, placebo-controlled trials of therapy have used histological staging to compare patient groups at entry into the studies, and a progression through the stages over time has been shown in most large series, yet with a marked individual variation[20]. One cyclosporin trial showed slowing down of disease progression as assessed by staging[21], but this was not confirmed in a larger study testing the same drug[22]. Recently, Locke *et al.*[23], using the Markov statistical model on stagings of yearly repeat biopsies from previous treatment trials, found that a majority of patients with stage 1–3 PBC will progress histologically within two years. They suggest that the time course of histological progression as demonstrated in their series may be helpful in determining number of patients and length of time necessary to appreciate a treatment effect in future therapy trials.

In addition to staging, a number of histological parameters have been assessed and scored in sequential biopsy specimens that have arisen in various multicentre trials. Severe porto–portal bridging fibrosis has been shown to correlate inversely with survival[23]; the presence of cirrhosis and perivenular cholestasis independently implied a poor prognosis[24,25]; and, in a large series of sequential biopsies, cirrhosis with extensive cholestasis, prominent Mallory's hyalines and halo formation, was more common in specimens taken within two years of death[20]. However, in most instances, multivariate analysis has failed to show significant effect of treatment on any histological parameter. The aberrant expression of HLA-class I on liver cells in PBC has been shown to be reduced by ursodeoxycholic acid (UDCA) therapy[26], but further studies are needed to confirm if change in class I expression can be a marker of treatment efficacy in PBC. Difficulties in selecting histological parameters to be scored arise from the fact that florid bile duct damage, the cornerstone of early stages of PBC, is only sampled in some 50% of needle biopsy specimens from PBC; in addition tissue damage usually evolves from a cellular, probably immunologically mediated, mechanism (destructive cholangitis and lymphocytic piecemeal necrosis) to a chemically induced injury secondary to impaired bile flow and hydrophobic bile salt retention (biliary piecemeal necrosis with cholate-static changes)[20]. Recent drug trials have move from the traditional repeat histology to using clinical symptoms and biochemical parameters for assessing treatment efficacy[27,28]. UDCA has been shown to improve serum bilirubin, liver enzymes and symptoms. Given its potential mechanism of action, UDCA is bound to have some effect on the cholate-static changes present at the porto–parenchymal interface, but this and the long-term effect on histology have to be demonstrated, a task which may well be difficult due to ethical considerations.

Primary sclerosing cholangitis

The patchy nature of hepatic damage and the variable sizes of affected bile ducts in primary sclerosing cholangitis (PSC), make biopsy even more difficult to interpret than in PBC. The degree of ductopenia shows a marked individual variation, is difficult to quantify, and inconsistent episodes of superimposed cholangitis may complicate the histological picture. Nevertheless, the same histological staging system as that used for PBC is applicable and has been shown to be an independent prognostic factor in at least two large studies on the natural history of PSC[29,30]. Several clinical trial of UDCA have resulted in an improvement of symptoms, cholestasis and hepatocytolysis enzyme markers, and even in predicted mortality in PSC. Two placebo-controlled studies measured histological parameters: one showed some improvement, particularly in the degree of portal inflammation[31]; the other reported a significant improvement in histopathology evaluated by multiparametric scores, as well as a marked reduction in HLA class I molecule expression[32] in the treated groups. O'Brien *et al.*[33], in a 30-month study reporting the persistence of beneficial effects and relapse after treatment withdrawal, advocate initiation of a larger clinical trial with serial morphological evaluations of the liver and biliary tree.

References

1. Scheuer PJ. Classification of chronic viral hepatitis: A need for reassessment. J Hepatol. 1991;13:372–4.
2. Gerber M. Chronic hepatitis C: Beginning of the end of a time-honoured nomenclature. Hepatology. 1992;15:733–4.

3. Zetterman RK. Chronic hepatitis: Is it persistent, active, or just chronic. Am J Gastroenterol. 1993;88:1–2.
4. Ludwig J. Histopathological diagnosis and terminology of chronic hepatitis. J Hepatol. 1995;23(Suppl 1):49–53.
5. De Groote J, Desmet V, Gedigk P *et al.* A classification of chronic active hepatitis. Lancet. 1968;ii:626–82.
6. Desmet VJ, Gerber M, Hoofnagle JH, Manns M, Scheuer PJ. Classification of chronic hepatitis: Diagnosis, grading, and staging. Hepatology. 1994;19:1513–20.
7. Ishak KG. Chronic hepatitis. Morphology and nomenclature. Modern Pathol. 7:690–713.
8. International Working Party. Terminology of chronic hepatitis. Am J Gastroenterol. 1995;90:181–9.
9. Theodossi A, Skene AM, Portmann B *et al.* Observer variation in assessment of liver biopsies including analysis by kappa statistic. Gastroenterology. 1980;79:232–41.
10. Knodell RG, Ishak KG, Black WC *et al.* Formulation and application of a numerical scoring system for assessing histological activity in asymptomatic chronic active hepatitis. Hepatology. 1981;1:431–5.
11. Bedossa P, Bioulac-Sage P, Callard P *et al.* Intraobserver variations in liver biopsy interpretation in patients with chronic hepatitis C. Hepatology. 1994;20:15–20.
12. Lok ASF, Lindsay I, Scheuer PJ, Thomas HC. Clinical and histological features of delta infection in chronic hepatitis B virus carriers. J Clin Pathol. 1985;38:530–3.
13. Bianchi L, Gudat F. Chronic hepatitis. *In*: MacSween RNM, Anthony PP, Scheuer PJ, Burt A, Portmann B, editors. Pathology of the liver, 3rd edition. Edinburgh: Churchill Livingstone, 1995:349–65.
14. Goldin R, Patel N, Goldin J *et al.* Comparison of liver biopsies in chronic hepatitis: Knodell or Scheuer? J Pathol. 1993;169:S10.
15. Banner BF, Barton AL, Cable EE, Smith L, Bonkovsky HL. A detailed analysis of the Knodell score and other histologic parameters as predictors of response to interferon therapy in chronic hepatitis C. Mod Pathol. 1995;8:232–8.
16. International Group. Histological grading and staging of chronic hepatitis. J Hepatol. 1995;22:696–9.
17. Rubin E, Schaffner F, Popper H. Primary biliary cirrhosis. Chronic non-suppurative destructive cholangitis. Am J Pathol. 1965;46:387–407.
18. Scheuer PJ. Primary biliary cirrhosis. Proc R Soc Med. 1967;60:1257–60.
19. Ludwig J, Dickson ER, MacDonald GSA. Staging of chronic non-suppurative destructive cholangitis (syndrome of primary biliary cirrhosis). Virchows Arch [A]. 1978;379–92.
20. Portmann B, Popper H, Neuberger J, Williams R. Sequential and diagnostic features in primary biliary cirrhosis based on serial histologic studies in 209 patients. Gastroenterology. 1985;88:1777–90.
21. Wiesner RH, Ludwig J, Lindor KD *et al.* A controlled trial of cyclosporine in the treatment of primary biliary cirrhosis. N Engl J Med. 1990;322:1419–24.
22. Lombard M, Portmann B, Neuberger J *et al.* Cyclosporin A treatment in primary biliary cirrhosis: Results of a long-term placebo controlled trial. Gastroenterology. 1993; 104:519–26.
23. Locke GR, Therneau TM, Ludwig J, Dickson ER, Lindor KD. Time course of histologic progression in primary biliary cirrhosis. Hepatology (in press).
24. Roll J, Boyer JL, Barry D, Klatskin G. The prognostic importance of the clinical and histological features in primary biliary cirrhosis. N Engl J Med. 1983;308:1–7.
25. Mahl TC, Shockcor W, Boyer JL. Primary biliary cirrhosis: Survival of a large cohort of symptomatic and asymptomatic patients followed for 24 years. J Hepatol. 1994;20:707–13.
26. Calmus Y, Gane P, Rouger P, Poupon R. Hepatic expression of class I and class II histocompatibility complex molecules in primary biliary cirrhosis. Hepatology. 1990;11:12–5.
27. Poupon RE, Poupon R, Balkau B, and the UDCA-PBC Study. Ursodiol for the longterm treatment of primary biliary cirrhosis. N Engl J Med. 1994;330:1342–7.
28. Poupon RE, Chretien Y, Poupon R, Paumgartner G. Serum bile acids in primary biliary cirrhosis: Effect of ursodeoxycholic acid therapy. Hepatology. 1993;17:599–604.
29. Wiesner RH, Grambsch PM, Dickson ER *et al.* Primary sclerosing cholangitis: Natural history, prognostic factors and survival analysis. Hepatology. 1989;10:430–6.
30. Farrant M, Hayllar KM, Wilkinson ML *et al.* Natural history and prognostic variables in primary sclerosing cholangitis. Gastroenterology. 1991;100:1710–7.

31. Stiehl A, Walker S, Stiehl L *et al.* Effect of ursodeoxycholic acid on liver and bile duct disease in primary sclerosing cholangitis. A 3-year pilot study with a placebo-controlled study period. J Hepatol. 1994;20:57–64.
32. Beuers U, Spengler U, Kruis W *et al.* Ursodeoxycholic acid for treatment of primary sclerosing cholangitis: A placebo-controlled trial. Hepatology. 1992;16:707–14.
33. O'Brien CB, Senior JR, Arora-Mirchandani R, Batta AK, Salen G. Ursodeoxycholic acid for the treatment of primary sclerosing cholangitis: A 30-month pilot study. Hepatology. 1991;14:838–47.

15
Measurement of quality of life

A. J. CHWALOW

INTRODUCTION

Health care has recently tended to take a more global perspective when considering the individual patient. In addition to a measure of functional status, the integration of the disease into the daily life of the individual, or his quality of life, is now being evaluated. This concept, while relatively recent, is the result, in part, of changes in attitudes towards diagnosis and treatment of patients, particularly those with chronic and severe diseases. Over time, what is sought is a measurement of change in the level of well-being during the evolution of an illness. In clinical trials, the different levels that exist between two groups may be measured.

While some authors suggest that if quality of life as an endpoint is not shown to be improved, the patient should not be treated[1], this is still considered to be an extreme position. As the sensitivity or responsitivity of most scales is still being studied, this measurement tool should not be considered as a surrogate measure, but rather as a complementary one.

Rigorous validation of a quality of life scale requires both a qualitative and a quantitative approach, with attention being paid to the methodological issues in scale development. Specific statistical techniques are used to modify evolving versions. The cross-cultural adaptation of an existing scale into another language requires a rigorous qualitative phase before the quantitative phase is begun. The end product of this approach should be an equivalent scale, rather than a literal translation. While, for the most part, scales have been developed in Anglo-Saxon cultures and then translated and more or less validated in other cultures, the problems with cross-cultural validation are beginning to be addressed by those working in the field. Cultural anthropologists have described differences in expectations, social relationships, life styles, etc., all of which could have an effect on perceptions of the impact of the illness on quality of life.

BACKGROUND

It is well-known that chronic diseases, such as hepatic and other gastrointestinal diseases, have an effect on all aspects of daily life. There are three dimensions that, when combined, comprise the currently accepted measure of Health Related Quality of Life (HRQOL): psychological, social and functional.

Historically, clinicians have first developed a series of functional measures, associated with a specific pathology. However, it would seem obvious that the inclusion of psychological and social dimensions is essential in any estimate of prognosis. In addition to a measure of functional status, the integration of the disease into the daily life of the individual must be evaluated. The assessment of chronic diseases has forced the development of scales that measure all three of these dimensions[2], both objectively and subjectively. These scales can be used to:

- help monitor the results of care in combination with clinical measures;
- quantify change in health status over time;
- contribute to a better understanding of the patient's point of view;
- predict future outcomes;
- facilitate communication among those responsible for policy decisions; and
- assist in the development of health interventions[3,4].

Each scale has a specific measurement objective. A revue of the existing scales shows differences in the scope of the aspects measured. Certain scales have been constructed to measure a single aspect of health status[5–10], while others, more global in nature, assess the three elements necessary for a measure of quality of life[11–15]. Whether a generic or a disease specific scale is used depends on the ultimate objectives of the investigators and the sensitivity of the measurements used.

In gastroenterology, emphasis is now being placed on liver diseases[16–21], rather than solely on intestinal problems[22–24]. Few studies, however, in hepatology, have used standardized, validated scales to measure quality of life[16,17]. Most rely on qualitative assessments specific to the population being studied[18–21]. This eliminates the possibility of making comparisons between different populations or standardizing quality of life as an endpoint.

METHODOLOGICAL ISSUES

No matter which dimension is being evaluated, it is absolutely necessary that the measure meets the methodological criteria demanded of all measurement tools[25], i.e. is it valid, and does it measure what it is intended to measure?

Validity

Validity is the ability of the scale to measure what it is supposed to measure. As there is no absolute standard (content validity) against which to compare this measure for quality of life, other types of validity are used:

1. Construct validity: Do scale items or observations reflect the dimension being tested as defined by experts? Is there a theoretical judgement by the experts on the structure of the scale?
2. Face validity: Refers to the understanding and acceptance of the questionnaire by the subjects themselves. What do they think the scale is measuring?

Do they understand the questions? Can they find themselves in the items and the responses?

3. Concurrent validity: Asks if the scale is correlated with other concurrent variables, e.g. does quality of life worsen as the disease progresses?
4. Predictive validity: Does the scale predict other variables, e.g. is a worse level of quality of life predictive of an earlier mortality rate?

Reliability

Reliability is a fundamental aspect of validity. In scaling, reliability generally refers to the internal consistency of the scale developed; do the items hang together, are they measuring the same factor[4,26,27]? A scale is reliable if it gives comparable results in comparable situations. There are three basic types of reliability:

1. Test-retest correlation coefficients are two observations of the same subject at two different times, assuming that his/her status is stable.
2. Coefficient of kappa is a statistical test that correlates two different observers of the same subject at the same time.
3. Internal consistency is determined with a single administration of the scale. It reflects the internal homogeneity of the items in the scale in that they measure the same dimensions. A number of different indicators can be used, but the coefficient of Cronbach's alpha is the most frequent.

Sensitivity and specificity

As with all measures the scales must be both sensitive and specific. The scale is sensitive if it differentiates one individual from another. The lower the rate of *false negatives*, the more *sensitive* the test. A scale is specific if it varies only with the observation it is intended to measure. The lower the rate of *false positives*, the more *specific* the test. The validity coefficient cannot *exceed* the reliability coefficient, hence the lower the reliability, the lower the validity. Note, however, that high reliability does *not* ensure high validity.

Scale administration

The method of scale administration is often a critical factor in whether or not quality of life can be measured. Often the amount of resources available determines if the scale will be done as a self-administered questionnaire or an interview. With a self-administered scale the subject fills out a questionnaire, under standardized conditions, after having received instructions. The advantages of this method are that the questionnaire can be administered by a lay person, its utilization is simple and may be repeated as many times as necessary, and there is no interviewer distortion. There are, however, disadvantages as well. The subject must be able to read and write and any distortion due to misinterpretation cannot be corrected. The respondent may be influenced by a desire to please the person doing the study and there may be systematic or response biases that go unnoticed. When the scale is administered using an interviewer, the interviewer completes the questionnaire. It is understood that the interviewer must be trained and that if more than one interviewer is used, the inter-interviewer reliability must be tested. This type of method allows for an evaluation that is standardized and uniform regardless of the subject or the circumstances. All questions are posed in the same fashion, therefore eliminating the bias found in the classic open-ended interview.

Types of responses

Measurement scales are usually divided by the types of responses that they allow. Dichotomous or nominal level responses such as yes/no, present/absent are generally the simplest types of scales and are the easiest to administer in unsophisticated populations. The Sickness Impact Profile[13] and the Nottingham Health Profile[14] are examples of generic quality of life scales using this format. Occasionally, the notion of doubt or degree is introduced, i.e. yes/no/maybe, raising the scale to the ordinal level.

When scales have multiple alternative responses, they are said to be interval. Adverbs indicate the frequency or intensity of the responses (always, sometimes, never). Differences must represent equal intervals between the responses which is often a problem in the construction of new scales. Unipolar items are those where one end of the interval level scale represents a normal state, i.e. no pain to very painful. Bipolar items, on the other hand, are those where the normal state falls in the middle of the scale, i.e. manic to depressed. An equal number of intervals reduces the tendency of regression towards the mean. Some scales are presented graphically, i.e. visual analog scales (10 cm).

Calculation of the global score

The calculation of the global score can be done by a simple sum of the values attributed to the items. This is frequently used and very effective. Many more sophisticated scales use an estimate of the weight of each of the items. Weighting is obtained by using a principal component factor analysis or a pilot study in a representative group of subjects, asking them to give relative weights to the items. Both approaches have their defenders and the resulting weights are often a compromise between the two methods. Weighting can be especially important in cross-cultural evaluation as different cultures place different values on the severity of the evolution of the disease.

CONCLUSIONS AND QUESTIONS

By definition, quality of life takes into account all dimensions of the individual. Scales should be able to assess the importance that each individual attaches to different facets of his life. The scale must be able to appreciate the level of well-being associated with events related to chronic disease, without reducing the integrated concept of quality of life to that of quality of health. These measures are necessary if the subjective importance that the patient attaches to his health status is to play any role in the decisions made by health care providers.

Are we trying to quantify the unquantifiable? If we keep in mind that the intent is to measure a difference over time or between two groups, without giving any intrinsic value to that difference, the goal would seem to be both possible and desirable. We must accept, however, that the concept of an absolute standard is unnecessary as the interest is in comparability only.

Are there general axes that cross cultures? Only by attempting to develop comparable scales and assessing their relative importance in different cultures and languages will we be able to answer that question.

Why the current interest in quality of life? As stated in a recent editorial in *The Lancet*[28], for many diseases the increases in survival time are minimal and patient well-being is really the endpoint of interest. In addition, with the increase in lifespan and its concurrent increase in chronic disease, quality of life is a major issue for health care providers. It is incumbent, however, on those of us who try to use quality of life as a marker, to do it well and to address the issues that are relevant to patients rather than health care providers.

It is only in assessing the perceived impact of the illness on the patient's daily life, that an accurate measurement of the functional severity of the disease can be obtained. Such instruments allow for quantification and measurement of quality of life as a variable, and enable the comparison of the results of two or more separate measurements in one individual or in a group of individuals. These instruments are of value in comparative assessment of impact in groups or individuals, over time or at the same point in time.

Acknowledgement

Portions of the chapter were presented at the conference, 'Patient Education 2000', Geneva, June 1994 and published in Chwalow AJ. Cross-cultural validation of existing quality of life scales. *Patient Education and Counselling*. 1995;26:313–8.

References

1. Koopsmans PP. Registration of drugs for treating cancer and HIV infection: A plea to carry out phase 3 trials before admission to the market. Br Med J. 1995;310:1305–6.
2. World Health Organization. The ten years of the World Health Organization. Geneva: WHO, 1958.
3. Bell MJ, Bombardier C, Tugwell P. Measurements of functional status, quality of life, and utility in rheumatoid arthritis. *Arthritis Rheum*. 1990;33:591–601.
4. Ware JE. Standards for validating health measures: Definition and content. *J Chron Dis*. 1987;40:473–80.
5. Katz S, Ford AB, Moskiwitz RW, Jackson BA, Jaf MW. Studies of illness in the aged. The index of ADL: A standardised measure of biological and psychosomal function. *JAMA*. 1963;185:914–9.
6. Jette AM. Functional status index: Reliability of a chronic disease evaluative instrument. *Arch Phys Med Rehabil*. 1980;61:395–401.
7. Lee P, Jasani MK, Dick WC, Buchanan WW. Evaluation of a functional index in rheumatoid arthritis. *Scand J Rheumatol*. 1983;2:71–7.
8. Radloff LS. The CES-D scale. A self-report depression scale for research in the general population. *Appl Psychol Meas*. 1977;1:385–401.
9. Folstein MF, Folstein SE, McHugh PR. 'Mini-mental state': A practical method for grading the cognitive state of patients for the clinician. *J Psychiatr Res*. 1975;12:189–98.
10. Torrance G. Measurement of health status utilities for economic appraisal. *J Health Econ*. 1986;5:1–30.
11. Gerin P, Dazord A, Boissel JP, Hanauer MTh, Moleur P, Chauvin F. L'!evaluation de la qualité de la vie dans les essais thérapeutiques: Aspects conceptuels et présentation d'un questionnaire. *Therapie*. 1989;44:355–64.

12. Kaplan RM, Anderson JP. The quality of well-being scale: Rationale for a single quality of life index. In: Walker SR, Rosser RM, editors. Quality of life: Assessment and application. Lancaster, Boston, The Hague, Dordrecht: MTP Press Ltd, 1987.
13. Bergner M, Bobbitt RA, Carter WB, Gibson BS. The Sickness Impact Profile: Development and final revision of a health status measure. *Med Care*. 1981;19:787–804.
14. Hunt SM, McEwen J, Mc Kenna SP *et al.* The Nottingham Health Profile: Subjective health status and medical consultations. *Soc Sci Med.* 1981;15A:221–9.
15. Chambers LW, MacDonald LA, Tugwell P *et al.* The McMaster Health Index Questionnaire as a measure of quality of life for patients with rheumatoid arthritis. *J Rheum.* 1982;9:780–4.
16. Tarter RE, Switala J, Arria A, Plail J, Van Thiel D. Quality of life before and after orthotopic hepatic transplantation. *Arch Intern Med.* 1991;151:1521–6.
17. Abell TL, Cutts TF, Cooper T. Effect of cisapride therapy for severe dyspepsia on gastrointestinal symptoms and quality of life. *Scand J Gastroenterol.* 1993;28:60–4.
18. Wainwright SP. Recovery from liver transplantation – a literature review. *Adv Nurs.* 1994;20(5):861–9.
19. Lundgren M, Kristiansson M, Ericzon BG, Eleborg L. Improved quality of life after liver transplantation, *Transplant Proc.* 1994;26(3):1779.
20. Pennington JC. Quality of life following liver transplantation. *Transplant Proc.* 1989;21(3):3514–6.
21. Eid AE, Steffen R, Porayko MK *et al.* Beyond 1 year after liver transplantation. *Mayo Clin Proc.* 1989;64:446–50.
22. Dimenas E. Methodological aspects of evaluation of quality of life in upper gastrointestinal diseases. *Scand J Gastroenterol.* 1993;28 (Suppl. 199):18–21.
23. Dimenas E, Glise H, Hallerback B, Hernqvist H, Svedlund J, Wiklund I. Quality of life in patients with upper gastrointestinal symptoms – an improved evaluation of treatment regimens, *Scand J Gastroenterol.* 1993;28(8):681–7.
24. Morris PLP, Goldberg RJ. Validity of the 28-item general health questionnaire in hospitalized gastroenterology patients. *Psychosomatics.* 1989;30:290–5.
25. Chwalow AJ. Cross-cultural validation of existing quality of life scales. *Patient Education and Counseling.* 1995;26:313–8.
26. Cronbach LJ. Coefficient alpha and the internal structure of tests. *Psychometrika.* 1951;16:297–334.
27. Nunnally JC. Psychometric theory, 2nd ed. New York: McGraw-Hill, 1978.
28. Editorial. Quality of life and clinical trials. *Lancet.* 1995;346(8966):1–2.

16
Surrogate markers: quality of life in liver disease

H. U. FISCH, E. L. RENNER and C. R. B. JOYCE

INTRODUCTION

What is quality of life?

Physiological measurements and results of clinical trials provide relevant information to clinicians. However, particularly in chronic diseases, most measures are of limited interest to patients because they are often irrelevant to the patient's perception of well-being and its consequent effects on his or her social and psychological functioning. Patients, clinicians and health care providers are increasingly interested in assessing the effect of a treatment on both the pathophysiology and the perception of well-being by the patient. Obviously, the question of quality of life as a major surrogate marker is relevant in view of the socio-political importance of the problem. The prime goal should be, as always in quantitative science, to define quality of life in such a way that it can be reliably and validly measured.

Definitions of quality of life

In the last 30 years thousands of papers alleged to be about quality of life have been published making use of hundreds of definitions[1,2]. There is thus no universally accepted definition and no gold standard. There are many difficulties in comparing studies, particularly between various illnesses and treatment modalities.

As is not uncommon, an excellent description of the problem may be found in classic literature. 'When it comes to saying in what happiness consists, opinions differ, and the account given by the generality of mankind is not at all like that of the wise. The former take it to be something obvious and familiar, like pleasure or money or eminence ... Often the same person actually changes his opinion. When he falls ill he says that it is his health, and when he is hard up he has it that it is money' (Aristotle).

Modern alternatives are: 'Quality of life is what the patient says it is' or even 'Quality of life is not merely what the patient says it is, but what he tells himself or herself that it is'[3].

In spite of the bewildering array of definitions, there is general agreement that the essential set of dimensions of quality of life includes the subjective experience of physical, psychological and social function. Clearly, other dimensions can be added, such as social role activities, perceived influence of environmental factors, religious and/or spiritual dimensions. Sometimes it is difficult to distinguish between quality of life and psychiatric syndromes such as anxiety and depression. Anxiety and depression scales are in fact often included in composite measures of quality of life.

Reliability

Reliability estimates the consistency of the performance of an instrument used by different observers or different time periods. This essential information is not always available.

Validity

The question of validity is crucial. Most approaches rely on face validity, which examines whether an instrument *appears* to be measuring what it is designed to measure by its inventor. A somewhat more elaborate concept is that of content validity, which examines the extent to which the field of interest is sampled by the items of the scale.

TYPES OF QUALITY OF LIFE ASSESSMENT

Generic instruments versus disease-specific instruments

The most general method is the single question: how is your quality of life today? This gives neither detailed information, nor any notion of reliability. Some widely used instruments, such as the Sickness Impact Profile (SIP)[4], attempt to measure all relevant aspects of quality of life with the same questions, irrespective of the medical diagnosis of the patient. The SIP is a widely used health status measure, consisting of 136 questions scored in 13 categories: sleep and rest, emotional behaviour, body care and movement, home management, mobility, social interaction, ambulation, alertness behaviour, communication, recreation and pastimes, eating, work and the overall score. Generic instruments apply to many populations and may make possible broad comparisons of the impact of disease or treatment. Their disadvantage is that they may be unresponsive to changes, whether due to progress of the disease or beneficial or adverse effects of interventions.

Disease-specific instruments are intended to identify relevant changes in quality of life of patients suffering specific diseases. Their use in medical domains other than those for which they were intended is often unsatisfactory. An example is the use of the EORTC-QOL in liver disease[5].

Group versus individual

Quality of life instruments should assess the influence of all personal variables relevant to the subjective assessment of health status. In other words: quality of life is a state which each subject perceives individually. Clearly, this poses important methodological problems. The main problem of most approaches to quality of life is that they are intended to distinguish between groups or to assess change within groups of patients with the same disease. Because quality of life is such a highly individual matter the question may be raised whether a group approach is justified at all. New measures such as the Schedule for the Assessment of Individual Quality of Life (SEIQoL)[6,7], allow the quantitative assessment of individual quality of life.

Interview versus self-rating

The methods may be observational (a physician or other observer assesses the functional status of the patient) or they may be self-described. It is questionable whether quality of life can satisfactorily be observed by a third party.

REVIEW OF SELECTED PUBLISHED PAPERS ON THE EFFECT OF LIVER TRANSPLANTATION ON QUALITY OF LIFE

Almost all studies assessing quality of life in liver disease have focused on liver transplantation. The studies published in major English journals published since 1991 are briefly discussed below. Table 1 gives a summary of the designs and methods applied.

Adams *et al.*[8]: Employment after liver transplantation

The employment status and health status of 203 adult liver transplant recipients was assessed retrospectively using mailed questionnaires consisting of the SIP[4], the Medical Outcome Survey 36 items (MOS)[9], and an employment questionnaire. Employed patients had higher scores in the SIP and the MOS.

Bonsel *et al.*[10]: Assessment of the quality of life before and following liver transplantation

The authors studied 38 adult patients cross-sectionally and 14 patients longitudinally. They used the Nottingham Health Profile (NHP)[11]; the Karnofsky Index[12], a global one-item measure for health status, often used in oncological research; the Index of Well-Being[13], a global measure consisting of 11 items; the State–Trait Anxiety Inventory[14]; and the self-rating depression scale (SDS)[15]. Hepatic encephalopathy was assessed with the Child–Pugh classification. Only one patient showed clear signs of hepatic encephalopathy. In the longitudinal study (pre-transplant versus 3 months after transplantation), highly significant improvements were obtained in the NHP items energy and sleep, in the Karnofsky index, in the Index of Well-Being, and in physical complaints. Patients had significantly higher satisfaction with health, leisure time, daily activities and life as a whole.

Table 1 The effect of liver transplantation on quality of life

Author	*Design*	*No. of completers*	*Control*	*Hepatic evaluation*	*Subjective/ Objective*	*Assessment*	*Follow-up*
Bonsel *et al.*[10]	Cross-sectional Prospective	26 10–18	Waiting list	Child–Pugh	Interview Self-report	NHP Karnofsky Index of well-being STAI SDS	3 mo–10 yr
Collis *et al.*[16]	Cross-sectional Prospective	30	Population	Mini–Mental	Interview Self-report	CIS GHP NHP	3 mo–10 yr Weeks
Colonna *et al.*[19]	Retrospective	28	None			Ad hoc questionnaire	6 mo
Haagsma *et al.*[20]	Retrospective?	18	None		Interview	Not given	>5 yr
Kober *et al.*[21]	Cross-sectional Prospective	35 29	Normals Patients with chronic liver diseases		Self-report	EORTC STAI	36 mo
Leyendecker *et al.*[24]	Cross-sectional	45	Population		Self-report	GBB Ad hoc scale MSF ALL Index of well-being ACSA	9 mo

Table 1 Continued

Author	*Design*	*No. of completers*	*Control*	*Hepatic evaluation*	*Subjective/ Objective*	*Assessment*	*Follow-up*
Levy *et al.*[22]	Prospective	75				NIDDK	5 yr
Adams *et al.*[8]	Retrospective	203	None		Self-report	SIP MOS	>9 mo
Lowe *et al.*[29]	Cross-sectional	58	Matched controls		Self-report	NHP	>1 yr
Riether *et al.*[30]	Prospective	10		EEG Neuropsychology	Self-report Self-report Self-report Interview	BDI STAI SIP IMI	1 yr
Tarter *et al.*[36]	Prospective	130		Neuropsychology	Self-report	SIP	>2 yr
Tarter *et al.*[33]	Cross-sectional according to diagnosis	306			Self-report	SIP	
Tarter *et al.*[34]	Prospective	53	Normals		Self-report Interview	SIP SBAS	>2 yr

For explanations of the abbreviations see text

Collis *et al.*[16]: Psychiatric and social outcome of liver transplantation

Thirty consecutive patients were assessed, 2–21 weeks after transplantation, with the Clinical Interview Schedule (CIS)[17], a standardized psychiatric interview; the General Health Questionnaire (GHQ)[18]; and the NHP[11]. Mild anxiety, depression and impaired quality of life was found in some patients.

Colonna *et al.*[19]: The quality of survival after liver transplantation

The authors retrospectively assessed 28 adults and 32 children surviving more than six months after transplantation. An ad hoc questionnaire was used, containing questions on employment status, activity tolerance, frequency and duration of hospitalization, subjective determination of the quality of life, side-effects of medication and overall satisfaction. Adults were asked to compare their quality of life before liver transplantation and at the time of the survey. The results were very favourable towards liver transplantation and overall satisfaction was high.

Haagsma *et al.*[20]: Long-term results after liver transplantation in adults

Results were reported on 18 patients who survived for more than 5 years. Quality of life was good after transplantation. No methodological details were given.

Kober *et al.*[21]: A psychological support concept and quality of life research in a liver transplantation programme: an interdisciplinary multicentre study

Thirty-eight liver transplantation patients were compared cross-sectionally with a control group of patients with chronic liver disease and healthy individuals. In addition, 29 patients were followed longitudinally before and 2, 6, 12, 24 and 36 months after transplantation. Quality of life was assessed with the EORTC[5] and the Spielberg State–Trait Anxiety Inventory[14]. In the cross-sectional study, 38 patients who were successfully transplanted were compared with 12 outpatients with chronic liver disease (not specified) and 15 individuals. Patients with chronic liver disease had lower general well-being and social integration, and a higher level of anxiety than healthy volunteers. No difference was found in the overall quality of life between healthy subjects and successfully transplanted patients.

Levy *et al.*[22]: Quality of life improvements at one, two and five years after liver transplantation

The authors prospectively studied quality of life during evaluation for transplantation, and one, two and five years post-transplant. After 5 years, 79 patients of an original 213 pretransplant patients were still in the study. A complex questionnaire (National Institute of Arthritis, Diabetes, Digestive and Kidney Diseases quality of life form, NIDDK) was used. This questionnaire is composed of questions from the Karnofsky Performance Status Scale[23], the SIP[4], the Index of Well-Being[13], the MOS[9] and the NHP[11]. Originally, these questionnaires were administered by interviewers. The authors used a self-administered version. Quality of life improved in almost all of the many dimensions assessed.

Leyendecker *et al.*[24]: Quality of life of liver transplant recipients: A pilot study

In a cross-sectional study the quality of life of 45 transplanted patients was assessed 9 months after transplantation. An extensive self-rating test battery included: the Giessener Beschwerdebogen (GBB)[25], an ad hoc scale; Mehrdimensionaler Stimmungsfragebogen (MSF)[26]; an 'Alltag' Questionnaire (ALL)[27] which is supposed to measure ability to cope with everyday life; a German translation of the Psychological Well-Being Index; a questionnaire on Soziale Unterstuetzung[28]; and an anamnestic comparative self-assessment scale. Reference values were drawn from a general population. Patients complained more of exhaustion and suffered from more distress than the general population. Most measures of quality of life, however, were equal to those of one of the healthy control groups.

Lowe *et al.*[29]: Quality of life following liver transplantation: a preliminary report

The NHP[11] was mailed to 81 liver transplant recipients. Almost 50% had no problems with energy, pain, emotional reaction, sleep, social interaction and physical mobility. Data were compared with community based matched normals. The authors found a very high quality of life, similar to that for the same age and sex in the general population, in patients successfully transplanted.

Riether *et al.*[30]: Quality of life changes and psychiatric and neurocognitive outcome after heart and liver transplantation

In a prospective study both heart and liver transplantation patients were studied. The study started with 61 patients; after one year data on only 10 patients were reported. Psychiatric (Beck Depression Inventory (BDI)[31], STAI[14]) and quality of life self-ratings were used. In addition, the interpersonal styles (IMI, dominant, hostile, submissive, friendly[32]) were assessed before and after transplantation. EEG and an extensive neuropsychological battery were included. After 3, 6 and 12 months a significant improvement was found in most measures. Interestingly, candidates for OLT seemed both hostile and submissive towards the significant other, a pattern which was found unchanged 6 months after OLT. Neuropsychological values were normal one year after transplantation.

Tarter *et al.*[33]: Impact of liver disease on daily living in transplantation candidates

Differentiation between the aetiology of liver disease and its impact on handicap was attempted, using the SIP[4]. In general, the impact of disease on quality of life was relatively mild. Patients with primary biliary cirrhosis had the least, and patients with non-A-non-B-hepatitis the most severe impairment in quality of life. Another important finding was the absence of a relation between SIP score and severity of the Child Index. Similar to other chronic diseases, there was no clear-cut relation between the severity of the medical disease and the subjective handicap, as assessed by self-report.

Tarter *et al.*[34]: Quality of life before and after orthotopic hepatic transplantation

Fifty-three patients with chronic liver disease were studied before and at least two years after transplantation. Thirty-five normal volunteers served as controls. The social behaviour adjustment schedule (SBAS)[35] was administered as a semi-structured interview to an informant of the patient (either the parents or spouses of both patients and control subjects). The SBAS assesses social role performance and the burden placed on the family by the patient's illness. Improvement in behaviour, social role performance and burden due to the illness was observed. The SIP[4] was also used. Test-retest-scores reflected significant improvement across all health and psychosocial scales of the SIP. Compared with controls, however, certain scales of the SIP still indicated some, although clinically irrelevant, handicap. The authors concluded that liver transplantation is associated with substantial improvement in quality of life.

Tarter *et al.*[36]: Severity of hepatic encephalopathy before liver transplantation is associated with quality of life after transplantation

One-hundred-and-thirty patients underwent extensive neuropsychological testing before transplantation and completed the SIP[4]. At least 24 months after surgery the SIP was repeated. There was substantial improvement from pre-transplant to post-transplant quality of life. Interestingly, pre-transplant neuropsychological test scores explained up to 20% of the variance in magnitude of change due to the transplantation. The authors suggest caution in extrapolating these findings for the purposes of selection of transplantation candidates. The SIP scores at the post-transplantation assessment all approximated normality.

CONCLUSIONS

So far, the research in the impact of liver transplantation on quality of life is typical of the many problems faced by this new approach. In 13 studies examined, 21 different measures for quality of life were used. The design varied from uncontrolled clinical impression and retrospective comparisons to well designed prospective studies, and the time of observation was 3 months to 10 years. Interestingly, only 2 of the 13 studies took hepatic encephalopathy into account, an important, disease-specific variable. Indeed, in one of the large prospective studies[36], neuropsychological performance before liver transplantation explained up to 20% of the variance in quality of life. Since all published follow-up studies used an endpoint analysis, the apparent improvement of quality of life may be partially spurious, since the most sick patient or patients with complications may die. An intention to treat analysis would be more appropriate.

However, even if most studies suffer from methodological shortcomings, all agree that quality of life dramatically increases after liver transplantation. The message of these studies to both patients and health care providers is clear and unequivocal: liver transplantation is a worthwhile therapy for patients with end-stage liver disease.

References

1. Joyce CRB. Health status and quality of life: Which matters to the patient? J Cardiovasc Pharmacol. 1994;23(Suppl 3):26–33.
2. Joyce CRB. Psychosocial benefits. In: Walker SR, Asscher AW, editors. Medicine and risk-benefit decisions. Lancaster: MTP Press, 1987:99–107.
3. Joyce CRB. How can we measure individual quality of life? Schweiz Med Wochenschur. 1995;124:1921–6.
4. Bergener M, Bobbitt RA, Pollard WE *et al.* The Sickness Impact Profile: Validation of a health status measure. Med Care. 1976;14:57.
5. Aaronson NK, Ahmedzai S, Bernheim JL *et al.* Development of a core quality of life questionnaire for use in cancer clinical trials. EORTC Study Group of Quality of Life, Protocol 15861, 1986.
6. McGee HM, O'Boyle CA, Hickey A, O'Malley K, Joyce CRB. Assessing the quality of life of the individual: the SEIQoL with a healthy and a gastroenterology unit population. Psychol Med. 1991;21:749–59.
7. O'Boyle CA, McGee H, Hickey A, O'Malley K, Joyce CRB. Individual quality of life in patients undergoing hip replacement. Lancet. 1992;339:1088–91.
8. Adams PC, Ghent CN, Grant DR, Wall WJ. Employment after liver transplantation. Hepatology. 1995;21:140–4.
9. Stewart AL, Hays RD, Ware JE. The MOS short-form general health survey. Reliability and validity in a general population. Med Care. 1988;26:724–32.
10. Bonsel GJ, Essink-Bot ML, Klompmaker IJ, Slooff MJH. Assessment of the quality of life before and following liver transplantation. Transplantation. 1992;53:796–800.
11. Hunt SM, McEwen J, McKenna SP. Measuring health status. London: Croom Helm, 1986.
12. Grieco A, Long CJ. Investigating of the Karnofsky performance status as a measure of quality of life. Health Psychol. 1984;3:129.
13. Campbell A, Converse PE, Rodgers NL. The quality of American life. New York, NY: Russell Sage Foundation, 1976.
14. Spielberger CD, Gorsuch RL, Lushene RE, editors. STAI manual for the State–Trait Anxiety Inventory. Palo Alto, CA: Consulting Psychologists Press, 1970.
15. Zung WWK, Durham NC. A self-rating depression scale. Arch Gen Psychiat. 1965;13:63.
16. Collis I, Burroughs A, Rolles K, Lloyd G. Psychiatric and social outcome of liver transplantation. Br J Psychiat. 1995;166:521–4.
17. Goldberg D, Cooper B, Eastwood MR *et al.* A standardised psychiatric interview for use in community surveys. Br J Prevent Soc Med. 1970;24:18–23.
18. Goldberg D, Hillier VF. A scaled version of the general health questionnaire. Psychol Med. 1979;9:139–45.
19. Colonna J O II, Brems JJ, Hiatt JR *et al.* The quality of survival after liver transplantation. Transplant Proc. 1988;XX (1, Suppl 1):594–7.
20. Haagsma EB, Klompmaker IJ, Verwer R, Slooff MJH. Long-term results after liver-transplantation in adults. Scand J Gastroenterol. 1991;26 (Suppl 188):38–43.
21. Kober B, Küchler Th, Broelsch Ch, Kremer B, Henne-Bruns D. A psychological support concept and quality of life research in a liver transplantation program: An interdisciplinary multicenter study. Psychother Psychosom. 1990;54:117–31.
22. Levy MF, Jennings L, Abouljoud MS *et al.* Quality of life improvements at one, two and five years after liver transplantation. Transplantation. 1995;59:515–8.
23. Karnofsky DA, Burchenal JR. In: MacLeod E, editor. Evaluation of chemotherapeutic agents. New York: Columbia University Press, 1949:191.

24. Leyendecker B, Bartholomew U, Neuhaus R *et al.* Quality of life of liver transplant recipients. Transplantation. 1993;56:561–7.
25. Brähler E, Scheer J. Der Giessener Beschwerdebogen. Bern, Stuttgart, Wien: Huber, 1983.
26. Hecheltjen KG, Mertesdorf F. Entwicklung eines mehrdimensionalen Stimmungsfragebogens (MSF). Gruppendyn. 1973;2:110.
27. Gross M. Psychometrische eigenschaften zweier fragebogen zur erfassung der psychischen dimension der lebensqualität. In: Bullinger M, Ludwig M, Steinbüchel NV, editors. Lebensqualität bei kardiovaskulären erkrankungen. Göttingen, Toronto, Zürich: Hogrefe, 1991.
28. Bullinger M, Heinisch M, Ludwig M, Geier S. Skalen zur erfassung des wohlbefindens: Psychometrischeanalysen zum 'Profile of Modd States' (POMS) und zum 'Psychological General Wellbeing Index' (PGWI). Z Diff Diagn Psychol. 1990;11:53.
29. Lowe D, O'Grady JG, McEwen J, Williams R. Quality of life following liver transplantation: A preliminary report. J R Coll Gen Pract. 1990;24:43–6.
30. Riether AM, Smith SL, Lewison BJ, Cotsonis GA, Epstein CM. Quality-of-life changes and psychiatric and neurocognitive outcome after heart and liver transplantation. Transplantation. 1992;54:444–50.
31. Beck AT, Steer RA, Garbvin MG. Psychometric properties of the Beck Depression Inventory: Twenty-five years of evaluation. Clin Psychol Rev. 1988;8:77.
32. Kiesler DJ. Manual for the impact message inventory, research edition. Palo Alto, CA: Consulting Psychologists Press, 1985.
33. Tarter RE, Switala JA, Arria A, van Thiel DH. Impact of liver disease on daily living in transplantation candidates. J Clin Epidemiol. 1991;44:1079–83.
34. Tarter RE, Switala JA, Arria A, PlailR, van Thiel D. Quality of life before and after orthotopic hepatic transplantation. Arch Intern Med. 1991;151:1521–6.
35. Platt HS, Weyman A, Hirsch S, Hewett S. The Social Behavior Assessment Schedule (SBAS): Rationale, content, scoring and reliability of a new interview schedule. Soc Psychiat. 1980;15:43–55.
36. Tarter RE, Switala JA, Plail J, Havrilla J, van Thiel DH. Severity of hepatic encephalopathy before liver transplantation is associated with quality of life after transplantation. Arch Intern Med. 1992;152:2097–101.

Section V
Chronic Liver Diseases

17
Assessment of treatment in cholestasis

U. BEUERS and G. PAUMGARTNER

INTRODUCTION

Cholestasis is characterized by an impairment of bile flow and is observed in a wide variety of clinical syndromes. It may present as a transient rise of biochemical markers without clinical significance, but may also be the main feature of a number of chronic progressive liver diseases which finally lead to biliary cirrhosis, liver failure and death. This chapter will only relate to the second group of diseases and will focus on the most frequently observed chronic cholestatic liver diseases of the adult, primary biliary cirrhosis (PBC) and primary sclerosing cholangitis (PSC).

In these chronic cholestatic diseases, assessment of the disease-modifying potential of drugs has been difficult for a number of reasons:

1. *The aetiology of PBC and PSC is unknown.* Both diseases are induced by immunologic destruction of bile ducts. In PBC, florid asymmetric destructions of septal and interlobular bile ducts infiltrated and surrounded by dense accumulations of mononuclear cells are characteristic histologic features[1]. In PSC, less inflammation is typically observed in portal triads than in PBC, and concentric 'onionskin' layers of connective tissues surrounding intra- and extrahepatic bile ducts may be observed[2,3]. In both diseases, the bile duct damage may lead to retention of hydrophobic bile acids and other cholephils in the hepatocyte and the systemic circulation. This accumulation of potential toxins may mediate liver cell injury, apoptosis and necrosis. It may induce fibrosis and cirrhosis of the liver and may finally lead to liver failure and death. For the selection of appropriate patients to be included in therapeutic trials, it is important to realize that the pathologic changes observed in PBC and PSC may be reversible in the early phase of the diseases, when cholestasis is only mild and the majority of bile ducts are preserved. However, changes are irreversible in the late stage of disease once fibrosis has proceeded.
2. *The prevalence of PBC and PSC is low.* Estimates range from 3 to 15 per 100 000[1] and 1 to 6 per 100 000[3], respectively. These rates may

underestimate the real prevalence of both diseases since increasing numbers of asymptomatic patients are being diagnosed due to progress in diagnostic measures and greater awareness of these diseases by the medical community.

3. *PBC and PSC progress slowly and non-uniformly.* The median survival for a large cohort of patients with PBC diagnosed while symptomatic and followed for up to 24 years was 7.5 years[4], and it was 16 years for asymptomatic patients[4]. Asymptomatic patients as a group did not survive as long as a control population[4–6]. Patients with PSC show a remarkably similar course with median survival of 9 to 12 years from diagnosis and progressive disease in symptomatic as well as asymptomatic patients[3,7,8].
4. *A shortage of reliable prognostic markers* in both diseases makes a valid assessment of any new treatment modality difficult.
5. *Liver transplantation does not represent a reliable 'hard endpoint' for the assessment of treatment in cholestatic liver disease.* One of the 'endpoints' of these diseases, liver transplantation, is performed based on a variety of indications, not on only one well defined indication. The 'need for transplantation' may be judged differently from one centre to another. In addition, the time of liver transplantation depends not only on the need, but also on the availability of a donor organ.

In conclusion, the slow and variable progression as well as the low prevalence of PBC and PSC complicate the adequate assessment of any new treatment modality in these diseases. Thus, large cohorts of patients have to be studied for long periods of time using a very limited number of well evaluated 'endpoints' to achieve valuable conclusions.

ASSESSMENT OF TREATMENT IN CHOLESTASIS: GUIDELINES

For the adequate assessment of treatment in cholestatic liver disease, a number of guidelines have been proposed[9] which may be helpful for the appropriate design of controlled trials:

1. The rationale for treatment must appear convincing.
2. Adequate numbers of appropriate patients, including asymptomatic patients, should be studied.
3. Adequate duration of follow-up must be achieved.
4. A systematic bias in the results should be avoided by using:
   - a double-blind design;
   - the 'intent to treat' rule in data analysis; and
   - an objective guideline in deciding when to analyse and publish results.
5. Potential drug toxicities must be closely monitored.

A number of different medications such as azathioprine[10], chlorambucil[11], colchicine[12–16], corticosteroids[17], cyclosporin[18,19], methotrexate[20] and D-penicillamine[21–25] have been evaluated for the treatment of PBC and PSC during the last 20 years. However, neither immunosuppressive agents nor antifibrotic agents have convincingly been shown in controlled trials to be an effective and well tolerated treatment option.

Today, ursodeoxycholic acid (UDCA) is widely accepted as an effective and well tolerated treatment in PBC[26–30], and beneficial effects have also been observed in small groups of patients with PSC[31,32]. Liver transplantation is regarded as the treatment of choice in late stages of PBC and PSC[33,34]. However, it is important to note that the efficacy of these treatments as tested by trials following the guidelines mentioned above[9] and using the 'hard endpoint' of death has never been convincingly proven.

ASSESSMENT OF TREATMENT IN CHOLESTASIS: SURROGATE MARKERS

The efficacy of any treatment should ideally be proven by its beneficial effect on 'hard endpoints' in the disease under study which, for PBC and PSC, are death and, with the limitations outlined above, liver transplantation[35].

Since the low prevalence and the slow and variable progression of these diseases hardly allow detection of a potentially effective treatment by only using hard endpoints such as death or liver transplantation, a number of surrogate markers for prediction of prognosis have been studied. These surrogate markers, however, should fulfil two key criteria when used as prognostic markers for evaluation of treatment[35]. They should be of prognostic value in the disease under study; and should not be affected by the treatment under investigation.

Candidates for surrogate markers in chronic cholestatic liver disease include clinical signs and symptoms, biochemical tests, histological findings, prognostic scores and quantitative liver function tests.

Surrogate markers should be of prognostic value in the disease under study

Clinical signs and symptoms, biochemical tests and histological findings

A number of studies during the last 25 years have evaluated potential markers of prognosis in PBC, and, lately, also in PSC. Among these, clinical signs such as hepatomegaly, splenomegaly or ascites, symptoms such as pruritus or fatigue, biochemical markers such as serum levels of bilirubin, transaminases or alkaline phosphatase, and histological criteria were tested. Tables 1 and 2 summarize the results of the largest follow-up studies in PBC[10,36–42] and PSC[7,8,43]. In most of these studies, age represented an independent predictor of survival. This factor obviously cannot be modified by any treatment. In most studies, bilirubin proved to be a strong predictor of survival[7,10,36–43]. Fibrosis/cirrhosis was the histological criterion with the highest predictive power in those studies in which histological criteria were tested[7,8,10,36,39,41,43]. Interestingly, neither serum transaminases nor marker enzymes of cholestasis such as alkaline phosphatase were independent variables of prognosis in most of the studies.

Serum bilirubin has long been known as a potent predictor of survival in PBC[36,44,45]. In most patients, serum bilirubin levels increase very slowly for many years, and then rise sharply in the few years before death[45,46]. Based on

Table 1 Independent variables predictive of survival in PBC

Yale[36]	*European I*[10]	*Mayo*[37]	*Oslo*[38]	*Glasgow*[39]	*Australia*[40]	*European II*[41]	*Japan*[42]
Age	Age	Age		Age	Age	Age	Age
Bilirubin	Bilirubin	Bilirubin	Bilirubin	Bilirubin	Bilirubin	Bilirubin	Bilirubin
	Albumin	Albumin		Albumin	Albumin	Albumin	Albumin
		Prothrombin time				IgM	Cholesterol
Cirrhosis/ fibrosis	Cirrhosis			Fibrosis		Cirrhosis	
	Cholestasis			Cholestasis		Cholestasis	
				Mallory bodies			
Hepatomegaly	Oedema		Ascites		Ascites		
			Variceal bleeding	Variceal bleeding		GI bleeding	

Data from reference 34 (modified)

Table 2 Independent variables predictive of survival in PSC

Mayo[7]	*King's College*[8]	*Multicentre*[43]
Age	Age	Age
Bilirubin	Alkaline phosphatase	Bilirubin
Haemoglobin		
Histological stage	Histological stage	Histological stage
	Splenomegaly	Splenomegaly
	Hepatomegaly	
Inflammatory bowel disease		

Data from reference 34 (modified)

the data of Epstein *et al.*[45], Senior and O'Brien[46] proposed to approximate the expected time until death of a patient with PBC by using the simple equation:

$$\text{Serum bilirubin [mg/dl]} = 10/[\text{age at death} - \text{current age}].$$

This formula, however, has not been validated for the calculation of prognosis in patients with PBC, and cannot, therefore, be recommended for general use.

Thus, serum bilirubin is a good predictor of survival in chronic cholestatic liver disease[7,10,36–46]. However, serum bilirubin levels may be affected by extrahepatic factors, e.g. haemolysis or gastrointestinal bleeding. This indicates that use of a *single* variable for assessment of prognosis or assessment of any new form of treatment carries an inherent risk of incorrect prognosis.

Prognostic scores

In order to overcome the problem of incorrect prognosis by use of a single variable and to enhance the prognostic value of independent clinical variables predictive of survival, prognostic scores for the prediction of outcome in patients with chronic cholestatic liver disease were developed and validated by multivariate survival analysis using Cox's regression model[47].

Christensen *et al.* combined five variables which had been independently demonstrated by Cox multiple regression analysis to imply poor prognosis in PBC[10]. The 'European score', included age, bilirubin, albumin, and the histological criteria cirrhosis and central cholestasis. The practicability of this score, however, was limited because histological samples are not routinely available at each patient visit.

The Mayo model was the first prognostic score which did not require liver biopsy or other invasive procedures in the assessment of prognosis of patients with PBC[37]. All criteria – bilirubin, albumin, age, prothrombin time and oedema – were independent predictors of survival as demonstrated by Cox's proportional hazards multivariate regression analysis[37]. Using these parameters, expected survival of an individual patient could easily be calculated. The generalizability of the Mayo model was tested and confirmed by extramural cross-validation[48]. The Mayo risk score, therefore, should be part of any protocol for the assessment of a new treatment in primary biliary cirrhosis.

The precision of the Mayo score, like the former 'European score', is good for prognosis of groups of patients with PBC. However, it is not very precise for prognosis of an individual patient. This may partly be due to the fact that prognosis is based on data from just one time point during the course of disease and does not take follow-up data into consideration. Therefore, this score was labelled a time-fixed model[42]. One might argue that time-fixed models should not be used on follow-up data to obtain an updated prognosis which is needed for the assessment of any treatment[42].

To overcome this problem, Christensen *et al.* developed a time-dependent model by incorporating follow-up data[42]. This model ('European II', Tables 2,3) was based on data of 237 patients followed up regularly for up to 11 years and was validated in an independent group of 147 patients. The model allows calculation of short-term prognosis for the next 1 to 6 months. Prognosis may be calculated independent (A) or dependent (B) of histological findings, and death may be predicted unrelated (I) or related (II) to liver disease. Expected survival time may be easily calculated using pocket charts or a pocket calculator[42]. Therefore, the European risk score II should be included in the assessment of new treatment modalities in PBC.

In PSC, similar studies were performed by the Mayo Clinic and the King's College in London which included 174 and 126 patients, respectively[7,8]. Only age and histological stage were independent predictors of survival in both groups of patients (Table 2). The Mayo score, but not the King's College score was validated. Finally, a multicentre study on the natural history of PSC in 426 patients included the patients of the Mayo Clinic, King's College and those of three other centres[43]. The multicentre risk score revealed bilirubin, histological stage, age and splenomegaly as independent variables of survival (Table 2). This score was statistically validated. The multicentre risk score should be included in any protocol for the assessment of treatment in PSC.

Risk scores have been used for the estimation of survival in cohorts of patients with PBC as well as PSC at the time of liver transplantation[33,34]. Actuarial survival after liver transplantation as calculated by Kaplan Meier

Table 3 Prognostic scores for PBC and PSC

PBC	
Mayo model:	$R = 0.871 \times \log_e$ (bilirubin [mg/dl]) $- 2.53 \times \log_e$ (albumin [g/dl]) $+ 0.039 \times$ age $+ 2.380 \times \log_e$ (prothrombin time [sec]) $+ 0.859 \times$ oedema* (*0 = no oedema, no diuretics; 0.5 = oedema, no diuretics; or no oedema, but diuretics; 1 = oedema and diuretics)
European model:	$PI_{AI} = 2.530 \times$ [log (bilirubin [μmol/L]) $- 1.53$] $+ 1.39 \times$ ascites* $-$ $0.089 \times$ (albumin [g/L] $- 34.3$) $+ 0.04 \times$ (age $- 55$) $+ 0.65 \times$ gastrointestinal bleeding* (*0 = no, 1 = yes)
PSC	
Multicentre model:	$R = 0.535 \times \log_e$ (bilirubin [mg/dl]) $+ 0.486 \times$ histological stage* $+$ $0.041 \times$ age $+ 0.705 \times$ splenomegaly** (*1 = stage 1 and 2, 2 = stage 3, 4 = stage 4; **0 = no, 1 = yes)

survival analysis was markedly improved in these patients as compared to their expected survival without transplantation as calculated by the Mayo models for PBC and PSC, respectively[33,34]. This information is of interest because, for ethical reasons, the efficacy of liver transplantation in end stage cholestatic liver disease has never been validated in placebo-controlled trials.

Quantitative liver function tests

Valid data on the potential role of quantitative liver function tests as surrogate markers in cholestatic liver disease are limited. In a retrospective study on 61 patients with PBC, Reichen *et al.* showed that serial determination of galactose elimination capacity (GEC) predicted survival as well as the Mayo model did[49]. Death was expected in a patient when the galactose clearance was lower than or equal to 4 mg/kg/min. In this study, the time of death was predicted with an accuracy of 7±19 months using GEC. Prospective validation of these findings in an independent cohort of patients with PBC would strengthen the potential value of serial determination of quantitative liver function for the estimation of prognosis and the assessment of treatment in chronic cholestatic liver disease.

A role for indocyanine green clearance in prognosis of PBC has been claimed[50], but additional data have to be awaited. Other quantitative liver function tests such as the aminopyrine breath test or the MEGX test have not been studied prospectively in a serial fashion in patients with chronic cholestatic liver disease[51].

Candidate surrogate markers of fibrosis, hepatocellular injury and biliary secretion

Which tests or markers might be candidates for evaluation in the future? Besides the serial determination of quantitative liver function, markers of fibrosis such as hyaluronic acid, procollagen III aminopropeptide or laminin have high potential as valid surrogate markers (for details and references, see Chapter 12). In a group of PBC patients, hyaluronic acid and procollagen III aminopeptide were of prognostic value for the prediction of entry into the terminal phase of the disease[52]. In view of the key importance of fibrosis in the progression of PBC and PSC, serum markers of fibrosis should be included in any protocol for the assessment of treatment in chronic cholestatic liver disease.

The role of soluble intercellular adhesion molecule-1 (sICAM-1) as a surrogate marker in cholestatic liver disease remains to be determined since its prognostic value in PBC or PSC has not yet been established (for details, see Chapter 13).

Impairment of biliary secretion seems to be a key event for hepatocellular damage as well as the course and prognosis of chronic cholestatic liver disease. Therefore, determination of the biliary secretory capacity of the hepatocyte appears to be a valuable approach for the assessment of medical treatment in cholestatic liver disease. Colombo *et al.* have used ^{99m}TcHIDA for the measurement of hepatobiliary excretory function during UDCA treatment in patients with cystic fibrosis[53]. Jazrawi *et al.* have established ^{75}SeHCAT hepatic scintigraphy as a specific test of hepatic bile acid uptake and secretion[54]. Using this method, they were able to demonstrate improvement of biliary bile acid secretion in patients with PBC and PSC during UDCA treatment[55]. This methodological approach seems attractive, especially since the radiation exposure is comparatively low. Prospective evaluation of the prognostic value of this marker in chronic cholestatic liver disease would be of interest.

Surrogate markers should not be affected by the treatment under investigation

If one looks at routine parameters used to assess the efficacy of medical treatment in chronic cholestatic liver disease, many parameters used, such as serum transaminases or marker enzymes of cholestasis, are not suitable as surrogate markers because they are not of prognostic value in the disease under study. In contrast, serum bilirubin and liver histology have been clearly shown to be of prognostic value in PBC and PSC.

UDCA has been demonstrated to be an effective treatment in cholestatic liver disease in a number of studies[26–32]. Secretion of bilirubin into bile, however, has been demonstrated in experimental models to be stimulated by bile acids, indicating a potential interference of this marker with UDCA[35,56]. Is the improvement of serum bilirubin levels during UDCA treatment, as shown in a number of trials in PBC and PSC[26–32], explained only by interference of this marker with UDCA and unrelated to the mechanism of action of UDCA in cholestasis? This would mean that bilirubin, as well as any of the prognostic scores given in Table 3 – all are based on changes in serum bilirubin levels – may not be used for assessment of UDCA treatment in cholestatic liver disease.

Poupon *et al.* have recently shown that the prognosis of patients with PBC treated with UDCA for 4 years is improved when compared to those treated with placebo during the first 2 years and then switched to UDCA[30]. A meta-analysis of three large-scale trials has confirmed these findings[57] in line with the observed improvement of the prognostic marker bilirubin.

In addition, the major mechanism of action of UDCA in cholestatic liver disease, in our view, is the stimulation of hepatocellular secretion[58]. We have proposed a model of tauro-UDCA induced stimulation of hepatocellular secretion. This model implies Ca^{2+}-dependent stimulation of vesicle fusion with the canalicular membrane[58,59]. We[58] and others[60] speculate that UDCA may stimulate hepatocellular secretion mainly by inducing insertion of transport proteins into the canalicular membrane via stimulated vesicle fusion. Since bilirubin is transported across the canalicular membrane via a multispecific organic anion transporter, enhanced secretion of bilirubin during UDCA treatment may represent one feature of the beneficial effect of UDCA and may not only be explained by unrelated interference of bilirubin with the drug.

In line with this assumption, Kilmurry *et al.* reported that serum bilirubin and the Mayo risk score, which relies mainly on serum bilirubin levels, can still be used to predict prognosis in their patients when under UDCA treatment[61].

Further studies on the prognostic value of serum bilirubin levels and the prognostic scores (Table 3) in patients with PBC and PSC during UDCA treatment have to be awaited before a valid judgement on the use of these surrogate markers during UDCA treatment can be provided.

CONCLUSION

The assessment of treatment in cholestasis is complicated by the slow and variable progression and the low prevalence of chronic cholestatic liver diseases. It should rely on 'hard endpoints' such as death or, with the limitations outlined above, liver transplantation. Surrogate markers may facilitate evaluation of treatment. Their suitability, however, has to be vigorously validated.

References

1. Kaplan MM. Primary biliary cirrhosis. In: Schiff L and Schiff ER, editors. Diseases of the liver. Philadelphia: JB Lippincott, 1994:377–410.
2. Ludwig J, LaRusso NF, Wiesner RH. The syndrome of primary sclerosing cholangitis. Progr Liver Dis. 1990;9:555–66.
3. Lee YM, Kaplan MM. Primary sclerosing cholangitis. N Engl J Med. 1995;332:924–33.
4. Mahl TC, Shockcor W, Boyer JL. Primary biliary cirrhosis: Survival of a large cohort of symptomatic and asymptomatic patients followed for 24 years. J Hepatol. 1994;20:707–13.
5. Nyberg A, Lööf L. Primary biliary cirrhosis: Clinical features and outcome, with special reference to asymptomatic disease. Scand J Gastroenterol. 1989;24:57–64.
6. Balasubramaniam K, Grambsch PM, Wiesner RH *et al.* Diminished survival in asymptomatic primary biliary cirrhosis: A prospective study. Gastroenterology. 1990;98:1567–71.
7. Wiesner RH, Grambsch PM, Dickson ER *et al.* Primary sclerosing cholangitis: Natural history, prognostic factors and survival analysis. Hepatology. 1989;10:430–6.
8. Farrant JM, Hayllar KM, Wilkinson ML *et al.* Natural history and prognostic variables in primary sclerosing cholangitis. Gastroenterology. 1991;100:1710–7.
9. Wiesner RH, Grambsch PM, Lindor KD, *et al.* Clinical and statistical analyses of new and evolving therapies for primary biliary cirrhosis. Hepatology. 1988;8:668–76.
10. Christensen E, Neuberger J, Crowe J *et al.* Beneficial effect of azathioprine and prediction of prognosis in primary biliary cirrhosis: Model for decision making. Gastroenterology. 1985;89:1084–91.
11. Hoofnagle JH, Davis GL, Schafer DF *et al.* Randomized trial of chlorambucil for primary biliary cirrhosis. Gastroenterology. 1986;91:1327–434.
12. Bodenheimer H, Schaffner F, Pezzullo J. Evaluation of colchicine therapy in primary biliary cirrhosis. Gastroenterology. 1988;95:124–9.
13. Kaplan MM, Alling DW, Zimmerman HJ, *et al.* A prospective trial of colchicine for primary biliary cirrhosis. N Engl J Med. 1986;315:1448–54.
14. Warnes T, Smith A, Lee F *et al.* A controlled trial of colchicine in PBC: Trial design and preliminary report. J Hepatol. 1987;5:1–7.
15. Vuoristo M, Farkkila M, Karvonen A *et al.* A placebo controlled trial of treating primary biliary cirhosis with colchicine and ursodeoxycholic acid. Gastroenterology. 1995;108:1470–8.
16. Olsson R, Broomé U, Danielsson A *et al.* Colchicine treatment of primary sclerosing cholangitis. Gastroenterology. 1995;108:1199–203.
17. Mitchison HC, Bassendine MF, Malcolm A *et al.* A pilot, double-blind, controlled 1-year trial of prednisolone treatment in primary biliary cirrhosis: Hepatic improvement but greater bone loss. Hepatology. 1989;10:420–9.
18. Lombard M, Portmann B, Neuberger J *et al.* Cyclosporin A treatment in primary biliary cirrhosis: Results of a long-term placebo controlled trial. Gastroenterology. 1993;104:519–26.
19. Wiesner RH, Ludwig J, Lindor KD *et al.* A controlled trial of cyclosporine in the treatment of primary biliary cirrhosis. N Engl J Med. 1990;322:1419–24.
20. Knox TA, Kaplan MM. A double-blind controlled trial of oral-pulse methotrexate therapy in the treatment of primary sclerosing cholangitis. Gastroenterology. 1994;106:494–9.
21. Bodenheimer HC, Schaffner F, Sternlieb J *et al.* A prospective clinical trial of D-penicillamine in the treatment of primary biliary cirrhosis. Hepatology. 1985;5:1139–42.
22. Dickson ER, Fleming TR, Wiesner RH *et al.* Trial of D-penicillamine in advanced primary biliary cirrhosis. N Engl J Med. 1985;312:1011–5.
23. Neuberger J, Christensen F, Portmann B *et al.* Double-blind controlled trial of D-penicillamine in patients with primary biliary cirrhosis. Gut. 1985;26:114–9.

24. Matloff DS, Alpert E, Resnick RH, Kaplan MM. A prospective trial of D-penicillamine in primary biliary cirrhosis. N Engl J Med. 1987;316:319–26.
25. LaRusso NF, Wiesner RH, Ludwig J *et al.* Randomized trial of penicillamine in primary sclerosing cholangitis. Gastroenterology. 1988;95:1036–42.
26. Poupon RE, Balkau B, Eschwege E, Poupon R. A multicenter, controlled trial of ursodiol for the treatment of primary biliary cirrhosis. N Engl J Med. 1991;324:1548–54.
27. Heathcote EJ, Cauch-Dudek K, Walker V *et al.* The Canadian multicenter double-blind controlled trial of ursodeoxycholic acid in primary biliary cirrhosis. Hepatology. 1995;22:759–66.
28. Lindor KD, Dickson ER, Baldus WP *et al.* Ursodeoxycholic acid in the treatment of primary biliary cirrhosis. Gastroenterology. 1994;106:1284–90.
29. Combes B, Carithers RL, Maddrey WC *et al.* A randomized, double-blind, placebo-controlled trial of ursodeoxycholic acid in primary biliary cirrhosis. Hepatology. 1995;22:759–66.
30. Poupon RE, Poupon R, Balkau B. Ursodiol for the long-term treatment of primary biliary cirrhosis. N Engl J Med. 1994;330:1342–7.
31. Beuers U, Spengler U, Kruis W *et al.* Ursodeoxycholic acid for treatment of primary sclerosing cholangitis: A placebo-controlled trial. Hepatology. 1992;16:707–14.
32. Stiehl A, Walker S, Stiehl L *et al.* Effect of ursodeoxycholic acid on liver and bile duct disease in primary sclerosing cholangitis. A 3-year pilot study with a placebo-controlled study period. J Hepatol. 1994;20:57–64.
33. Markus BH, Dickson ER, Grambsch PM *et al.* Efficacy of liver transplantation in patients with primary biliary cirrhosis. N Engl J Med. 1989;320:1709–13.
34. Wiesner RH, Porayko MK, Dickson ER *et al.* Selection and timing of liver transplantation in primary biliary cirrhosis and primary sclerosing cholangitis. Hepatology. 1992;16:1290–9.
35. Reichen J. Pharmacologic treatment of cholestasis. Semin Liver Dis. 1993;13:302–15.
36. Roll J, Boyer JL, Barry D, Klatskin G. The prognostic importance of clinical and histologic features in asymptomatic and symptomatic primary biliary cirrhosis. N Engl J Med. 1983;308:1–7.
37. Dickson ER, Grambsch PM, Fleming TR *et al.* Prognosis in primary biliary cirrhosis: Model for decision making. Hepatology. 1989;10:1–7.
38. Rydning A, Schrumpf E, Abdelnoor M *et al.* Factors of prognostic importance in primary biliary cirrhosis. Scand J Gastroenterol. 1990;25:119–26.
39. Goudie BM, Burt AD, Macfarlane GC *et al.* Risk factors and prognosis in primary biliary cirrhosis. Am J Gastroenterol. 1989;84:713–6.
40. Jeffrey GP, Reed WA, Shilkin KB. Natural history and prognostic variables in primary biliary cirrhosis (abstract). Hepatology. 1990;12:A955.
41. Christensen E, Altman DG, Neuberger J *et al.* Updating prognosis in primary biliary cirrhosis using a time-dependent Cox regression model. Gastroenterology. 1993;105:1865–76.
42. Inoue K, Hirohara J, Nakano T *et al.* Prediction of prognosis of primary biliary cirrhosis in Japan. Liver. 1995;15:70–7.
43. Dickson ER, Murtaugh PA, Wiesner RH *et al.* Primary sclerosing cholangitis: Refinement and validation of survival models. Gastroenterology. 1992;103:1893–901.
44. Shapiro JM, Smith H, Schaffner F. Serum bilirubin: A prognostic factor in primary biliary cirrhosis. Gut. 1979;20:137–40.
45. Epstein O, Fraga E, Sherlock S. Importance of clinical staging for prognosis in primary biliary cirrhosis. Gut. 1985;26:A1126.
46. Senior JR, O'Brien CB. Mortality risk indices as outcome measures of the effectiveness of ursodeoxycholic acid treatment of cholestatic liver diseases. In: Paumgartner G, Stiehl A, Gerok W, editors. Bile acids as therapeutic agents. Dordrecht: Kluwer Academic; 1992:273–85.
47. Christensen E. Multivariate survival analysis using Cox's regression model. Hepatology. 1987;7:1346–58.
48. Grambsch PM, Dickson ER, Kaplan MM *et al.* Extramural cross-validation of the Mayo primary biliary cirrhosis survival model establishes its generalizability. Hepatology. 1989;10:846–50.
49. Reichen J, Widmer T, Cotting J. Accurate prediction of death by serial determination of the galactose elimination capacity in primary biliary cirrhosis – a comparison with the Mayo model. Hepatology. 1991;14:504–10.

50. Clements D, Elias E, Mc Master P. Preliminary study of indocyanine green clearance in primary biliary cirrhosis. Scand. J Gastroenterol. 1991;26:119–23.
51. Reichen J. Assessment of hepatic function with xenobiotics. Semin Liver Dis. 1995;15:189–201.
52. Poupon RE, Balkau B, Guéchot J, Heintzmann F. Predictive factors in ursodeoxycholic acid-treated patients with primary biliary cirrhosis: Role of serum markers of connective tissue. Hepatology. 1994;19:635–40.
53. Colombo C, Castellini RM, Balistreri WF *et al.* Scintigraphic documentation of an improvement in hepatobiliary excretory function after treatment with ursodeoxycholic acid in patients with cystic fibrosis and associated liver disease. Hepatology. 1992;15:677–84.
54. Jazrawi RP, Ferraris R, Bridges C *et al.* Kinetics of the synthetic bile acid ^{75}SeHCAT in man: Comparison with ^{14}C-taurocholate. Gastroenterology. 1988;95:164–9.
55. Jazrawi RP, de Caestecker JS, Goggin P *et al.* Kinetics of hepatic bile acid handling in cholestatic liver disease: Effect of ursodeoxycholic acid. Gastroenterology. 1994;5:373–81.
56. Goresky CA, Haddad HH, Kluger WS *et al.* The enhancement of maximal bilirubin excretion with taurocholate-induced increments in bile flow. Can J Physiol Pharmacol. 1974;52:389–403.
57. Heathcote EJ, Lindor KD, Poupon R *et al.* Combined analysis of French, American and Canadian randomized controlled trials of ursodeoxycholic acid therapy in primary biliary cirrhosis. Gastroenterology. 1995;108:A1082.
58. Beuers U, Nathanson MH, Isales CM, Boyer JL. Tauroursodeoxycholic acid stimulates hepatocellular exocytosis by mobilization of extracellular calcium, a mechanism defective in cholestasis. J Clin Invest. 1993;92:2984–93.
59. Beuers U, Nathanson MH, Boyer JL. Effects of tauroursodeoxycholic acid on Ca signals in isolated rat hepatocytes. Gastroenterology. 1993;104:604–12.
60. Häussinger D, Hallbrucker C, Saha N, Lang F, Gerok W. Cell volume and bile acid excretion. Biochem J. 1992;288:681–9.
61. Kilmurry MR, Cauch-Dudek K, O'Rourke K, Heathcote EJ. Is the Mayo model useful for predicting survival following the introduction of ursodeoxycholic acid treatment for primary biliary cirrhosis? Gastroenterology. 1995;108:A1097.

18
Hepatic uptake and excretion of bile acids: quantitative tests of liver function in chronic cholestatic liver diseases

R. P. JAZRAWI, A. G. LIM and T. C. NORTHFIELD

SURROGATE MARKERS: GENERAL CONSIDERATIONS

Surrogate markers of a disease are tests carried out in the short term that correlate with the long-term hard outcome measures of that disease. These tests can be useful in monitoring the prognosis and/or the effect of therapy. In general a good surrogate maker should fulfil the following criteria:

1. Measure a physiologically important process of the diseased organ in a quantitative way.
2. Be sensitive enough to detect changes in function at an early stage of disease.
3. Be both organ and disease specific (i.e. able to differentiate between diseases affecting the same organ.
4. Be carried out directly on the organ and describe a kinetic function.
5. Be non-invasive, thus enabling repeated measurements to be carried out for monitoring disease activity or effect of therapy.

Primary biliary cirrhosis (PBC) and primary sclerosing cholangitis (PSC) are chronic liver diseases characterized by cholestasis. Although their pathogenesis is not completely understood, the disease process (Figure 1) is thought to arise from an initial immunological insult targeted at the biliary epithelial cells, followed by further biliary and hepatic damage by the retained endogenous bile acids[1]. Ursodeoxycholic acid (UDCA) has been shown to improve liver function tests in both conditions[2]. One of the proposed mechanisms of action of UDCA is to increase hepatic excretion of endogenous bile acids and thereby reduce their intrahepatic retention[3]. On administration of UDCA, serum concentrations of endogenous hydrophobic bile acids fall[4]. Some investigators have also found enrichment of the UDCA pool at the expense of endogenous hydrophobic bile

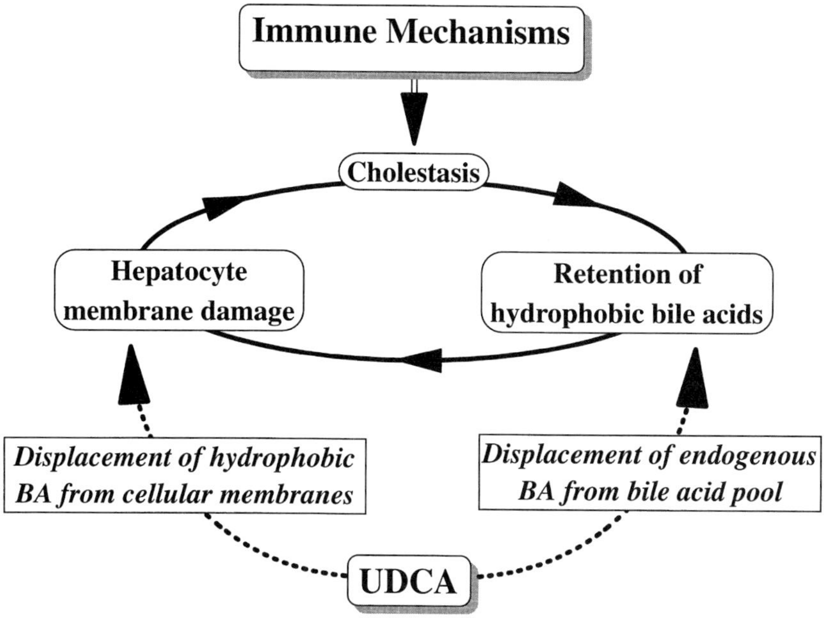

Fig. 1 Hypothetical illustration of the pathogenesis of PBC and the possible effect of UDCA therapy

acids, although this finding is disputed by others[5,6]. In PBC, UDCA may be clinically beneficial in the long term[7], but its benefit on hard outcome measures of the disease, such as death or need for transplantation, has not been demonstrated in a definitive way, despite the large clinical trials carried out[8–10]. This is because the majority of patients with PBC, particularly those with early stage of the disease, have long survival times and very low mortality in the short term.

It is well-known that bile acid handling is an integral physiological function of the liver and is therefore likely to be affected early in the course of liver disease. This effect is even more important in cholestatic liver diseases such as PBC, where by definition, bile flow impairment is one of the main characteristics of the disease process. Measurement of hepatic bile acid handling is therefore likely to provide a useful marker in liver disease. Until recently this has been carried out indirectly by assessing serum levels of bile acids. The introduction of the γ-labelled bile acid, ^{75}selenium-homo-taurocholate (^{75}SeHCAT), has made it possible for the first time to visualize the liver directly using γ-camera scintigraphy.

In this chapter, we shall first discuss briefly some of the surrogate markers currently used in PBC. We shall then describe the physiological properties of ^{75}SeHCAT by comparison with its naturally occurring counterpart taurocholic acid, and assess its suitability for measuring in a direct and quantitative way, physiologically important hepatic functions such as hepatic uptake and excretion of bile acids. Finally, we shall discuss the specific derangements in these functions and the effect of UDCA therapy in different cholestatic liver diseases.

SURROGATE MARKERS IN PBC

Several measurements have been proposed as short-term surrogate markers in PBC.

Conventional liver function tests such as serum levels of alkaline phosphatase and gamma glutamyl transpeptidase, are neither sensitive nor specific for PBC. They are indirect, as the measurements are carried out on serum and not on the liver. Thus they could be influenced by several diverse hepatic functions such as hepatic uptake and excretion, hepatic synthesis, hepatic transport and metabolism (conjugation etc.) and hepatic blood flow. Furthermore, many of these enzymes are also produced by other organs. Serum bilirubin level is considered to be one of the best prognostic indices in PBC, and is used in most prognostic scoring systems. However it is non-specific as it is also used in the prognostic scoring systems of most other liver diseases. It is also not a very sensitive marker as most patients with early PBC have normal serum bilirubin concentrations.

Liver biopsy is still the most widely used method for confirming the diagnosis of PBC as well as for staging of the disease, mainly because it is carried out directly on the liver. It is, however, invasive and not sensitive as it examines a minute fraction of the liver and is thus subject to gross sampling errors. This may be the reason why large multicentre trials[8–10], despite demonstrating some benefit on certain histological criteria, have failed to demonstrate a clear overall beneficial effect of UDCA therapy. Evidence regarding histological improvement on UDCA in PBC patients has, however, been reported following meta analysis carried out on several large clinical trials[11,12].

The effect of UDCA on certain dynamic physiological hepatic functions, such as the bromosulphthalein clearance test, aminopyrine breath tests and galactose elimination capacity has been assessed[13–15]. These studies have given conflicting results, probably because these tests are also indirect as they are not carried on the liver. They might therefore be influenced by similar factors affecting the conventional liver function tests (see above).

Other surrogate markers proposed for the assessment of disease activity and effect of UDCA therapy in cholestatic liver diseases include soluble serum adhesion molecules[16–18] and serum markers of fibrosis[19–21]. The clinical value of these markers is, however, not yet established.

PHYSIOLOGICAL PROPERTIES OF SEHCAT IN THE ENTEROHEPATIC CIRCULATION

^{75}SeHCAT is a synthetic analogue of the natural bile acid taurocholic acid, incorporating the γ-emitter ^{75}selenium in the side chain[22]. The word homo signifies that the molecular structure of the side chain is the mirror image of the natural bile acid. The fact that it is a bile acid makes it a potentially useful substance for assessment of physiological hepatic functions. The fact that it is γ-labelled makes it possible for the first time to carry out direct measurements on the liver.

Dynamics of SeHCAT in the enterohepatic circulation

^{75}SeHCAT has been shown to undergo enterohepatic circulation. Following oral administration of ^{75}SeHCAT to healthy subjects, activity starts to appear in the gallbladder within a mean of 60 minutes. After 24 hours, about 50% of the ^{75}SeHCAT detected in the abdomen is concentrated in the gallbladder in the fasting state[23]. This value is similar to the proportion of the bile acid pool stored in the fasting-state gallbladder[24]. Like natural bile acids, ^{75}SeHCAT is confined to the enterohepatic circulation, with <1% of the administered dose being detected outside the enterohepatic circulation at 4, 8 and 24 hours[25]. Following the simultaneous oral administration of ^{75}SeHCAT and ^{14}C-labelled cholic acid-taurine, Delhez *et al.*[26] found identical quantities of each of the two bile acids in stools collected over successive 24-hour periods for a period of 7 days.

The enterohepatic circulation as a whole can be assessed by measuring the fractional turnover rate for ^{75}SeHCAT by γ-camera scintigraphy over the gall-bladder area. This techniques assumes – as has been demonstrated[27] – that a constant proportion of the bile acid pool is stored in the gallbladder in the fasting state. In health, the overall fractional turnover rate for ^{75}SeHCAT[28] was found to be similar to that of the natural bile acid taurocholate measured by the classical Linstedt technique[29] (Figure 2).

Efficiency of intestinal absorption for SeHCAT

Several studies have measured the recovery of ^{75}SeHCAT in bile following oral administration. These studies provide indirect evidence that ^{75}SeHCAT is absorbed efficiently in the terminal ileum[25,30,31]. The first direct evidence came from studies by Galatola *et al.*[32]. They demonstrated that in healthy subjects, >95% of the administered dose of ^{75}SeHCAT was absorbed in one enterohepatic cycle[32] (Figure 3). Based on this and other studies[28,33], ^{75}SeHCAT was advocated as an ideal substance to test ileal absorption of bile acids.

Hepatic handling of SeHCAT

Following its oral administration both to rats with bile duct cannulae and to humans with a bile duct T-tube, Merrick *et al.*[30] demonstrated that more than 90% of the ^{75}SeHCAT activity was recovered in bile within 24 hours. Galatola *et al.*[32] demonstrated that following instillation distal to an occluding intestinal balloon, ^{75}SeHCAT recovery in bile collected proximal to the balloon, paralleled that of its natural counterpart, taurocholic acid. They concluded that both ileal absorption and hepatic handling of ^{75}SeHCAT were similar to those of the natural bile acid, taurocholate. In another study, Galatola *et al.* compared the serum kinetics for ^{75}SeHCAT with those of ^{14}C-taurocholate, using simultaneous scintigraphy and serial blood sampling in six non-liver disease patients[34]. The time activity course was very similar in all six individuals for ^{75}SeHCAT and ^{14}C-taurocholate. Initial and late plasma disappearance rates

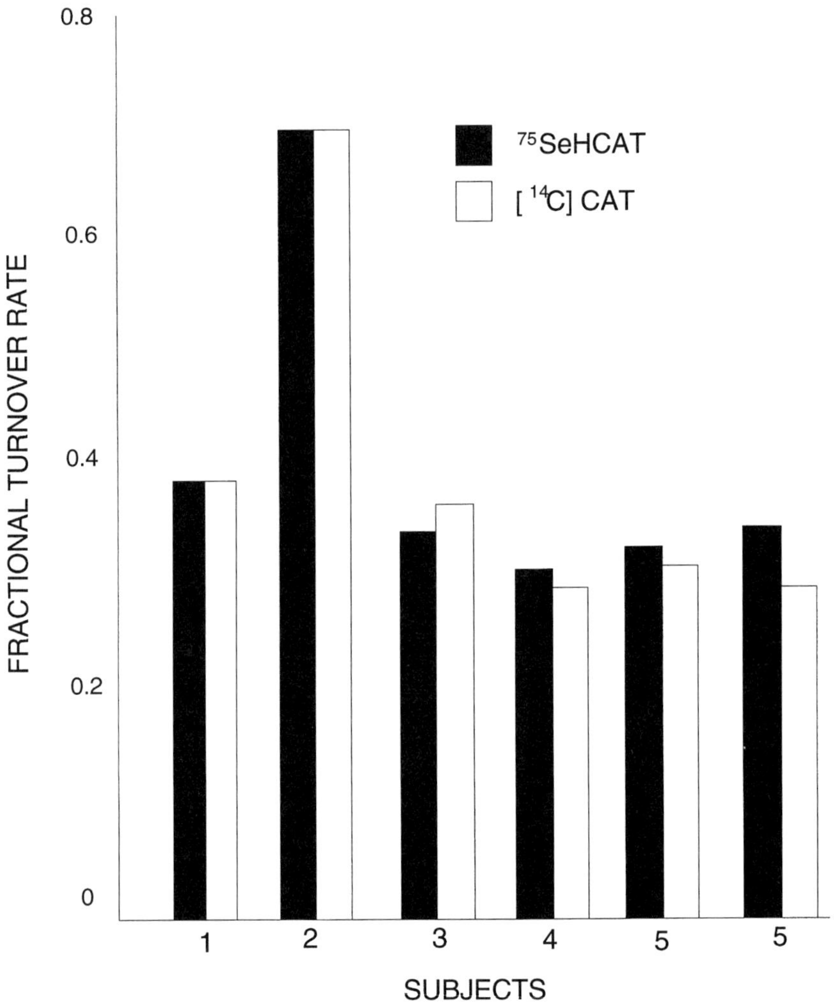

Fig. 2 Comparison of the fractional turnover rate for ^{75}SeHCAT and ^{14}C-taurocholate([^{14}C]CAT) in five healthy subjects. The study was repeated in subject 5 (reproduced from reference 28 with permission)

and plasma clearance were significantly lower for ^{75}SeHCAT compared to ^{14}C-taurocholate, probably as a result of the stronger protein binding of the natural bile acid[34]. However, the initial plasma disappearance of ^{75}SeHCAT could all be accounted for by its hepatic uptake, suggesting specific handling by the liver. This was not true for the hepatoscintigraphic γ-labelled agent, technetium^{99m} labelled hepatoiminodiactic acid (^{99m}TcHIDA). For ^{99m}TcHIDA, only half of the plasma disappearance was due to hepatic handling, the rest prob-

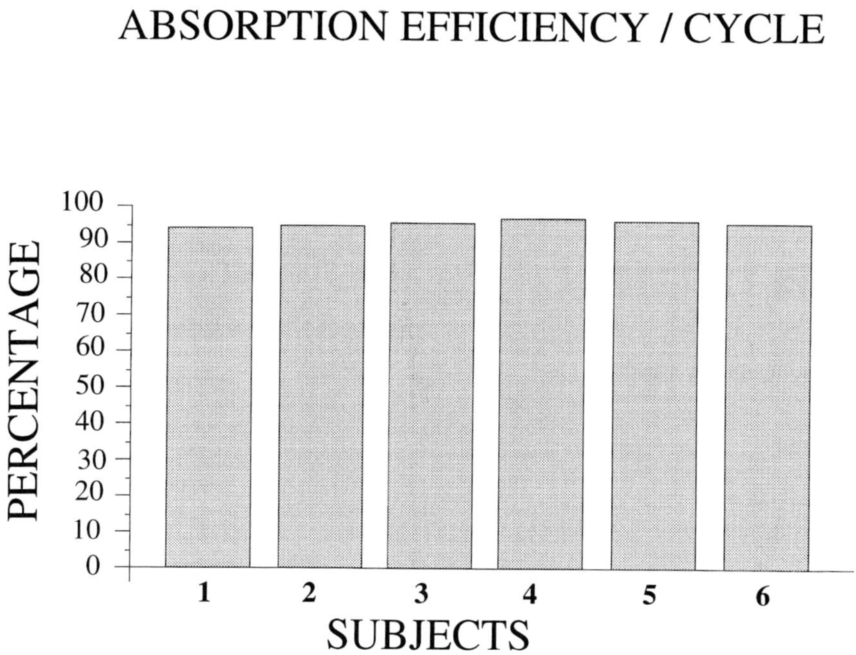

Fig. 3 First pass ileal clearance for ^{75}SeHCAT. In healthy subjects, >95% of the bile acid was absorbed per cycle

ably due to renal excretion (Figure 4). Furthermore, hepatic uptake, intrahepatic transit time and hepatic excretory rate were all more rapid for ^{75}SeHCAT than ^{99m}TcHIDA, suggesting a more sensitive handling of the bile acid by the liver[34].

Based on the physiological properties of ^{75}SeHCAT in the enterohepatic circulation in general, and on the sensitive and specific handling of ^{75}SeHCAT by the liver in particular, it is evident that measurement of hepatic uptake and excretion of bile acids using ^{75}SeHCAT, should provide a direct and quantitative test of liver function.

ANALYSIS OF HEPATIC BILE ACID UPTAKE AND EXCRETION USING SeHCAT

The methods and calculations involved for hepatoscintigraphic analysis of hepatic bile acid uptake and excretion have previously been described[34,35]. In brief, subjects were positioned under a large field of view γ-camera and injected with a bolus of ^{75}SeHCAT. Continuous γ-imaging is then performed over the liver, gallbladder, gut and heart areas. After correction for overlap, the following areas were used for analysis: liver alone, liver plus gallbladder, gallbladder alone and gallbladder plus gut. Hepatic uptake and excretory rates were

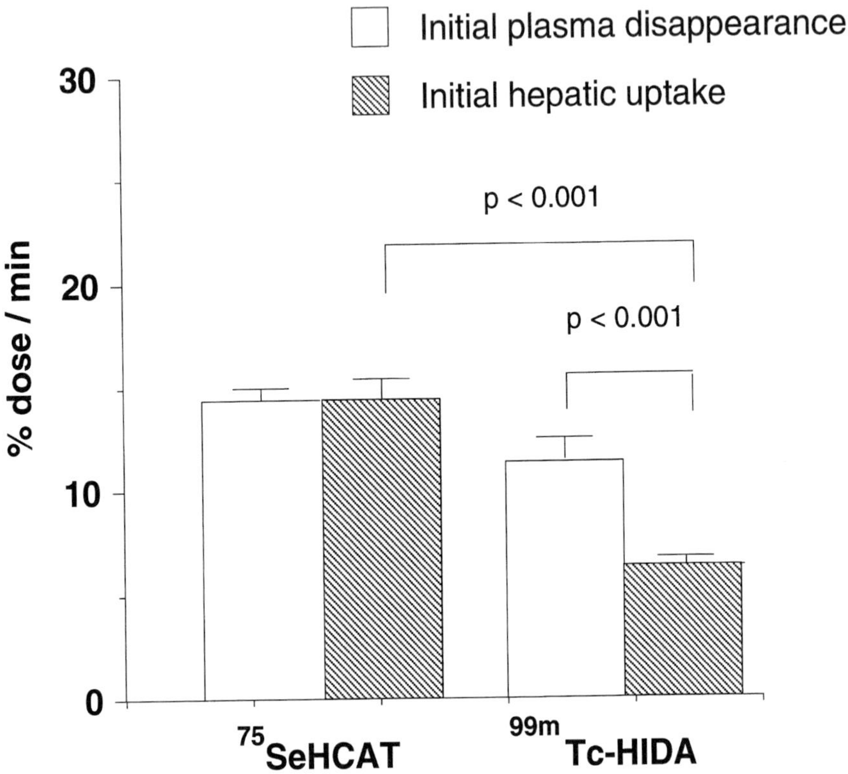

Fig. 4 Comparison of the mean hepatic uptake and plasma disappearance rates for ^{75}SeHCAT and ^{99m}TcHIDA in healthy subjects. For ^{75}SeHCAT but not ^{99m}TcHIDA, all the plasma disappearance rate could be accounted for by hepatic uptake, suggesting that the bile acid is handled more specifically by the liver

calculated and expressed as percent dose per minute. Hepatic transit time was taken as the time of first appearance of ^{75}SeHCAT activity in the gallbladder and/or gut. These, together with the time activity curve for ^{75}SeHCAT in a typical patient, are shown in Figure 5.

In both health and chronic liver diseases (PBC and PSC and other forms of cirrhosis), hepatic uptake and excretory functions do not correlate with each other, suggesting that they are separate and independent functions[35]. Hepatic excretory rate correlated with the levels of conventional serum markers of cholestatsis (alkaline phosphatase and γ-glutamyl transpeptidase) but not with markers of hepatocyte function (albumin and prothrombin time). Compared with controls, both PBC and PSC show defects in the excretory rather than the uptake phase of hepatic bile acid handling, indicating bile acid retention within the liver[35]. PBC patients with histologically more advanced disease had significantly lower hepatic excretory and uptake rate[35].

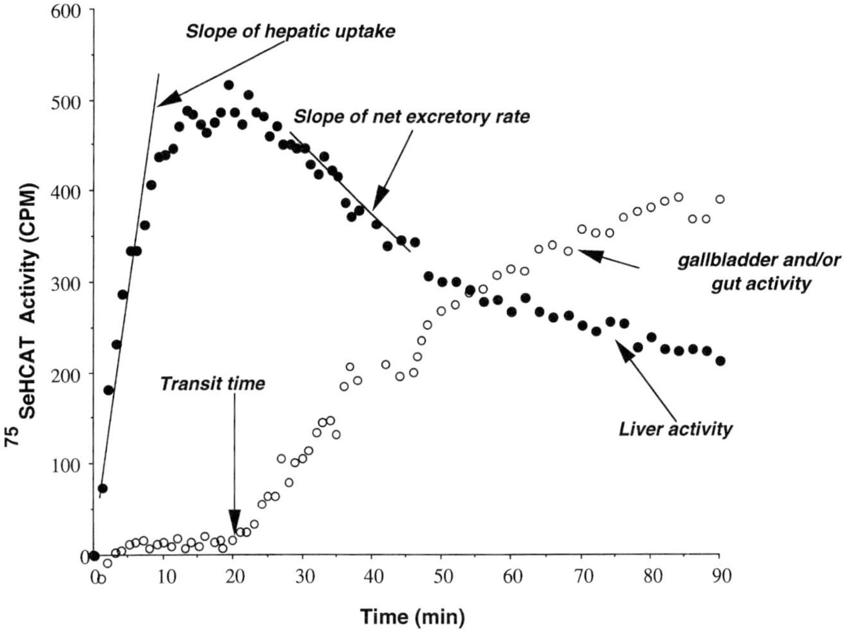

Fig. 5 Time activity (cpm) for ^{75}SeHCAT in a typical patient during the 90-minute study period. The slopes for increase and decrease in ^{75}SeHCAT activity over the liver area of interest were used for measuring uptake and excretion. Transit time is also shown over the gallbladder + gut area of interest (reproduced from reference 35 with permission)

UDCA AND HEPATIC BILE ACID UPTAKE AND EXCRETION

We have applied this new methodology in determining the effect of treatment of PBC and PSC with UDCA[35]. We studied 12 PBC patients and 5 PSC patients before and after 3 months of treatment with UDCA at a dose of 10 mg/kg/day. UDCA had no effect on initial hepatic uptake rate during UDCA (NS). However, significant improvements were found in transit time ($p<0.001$), net hepatic excretory rate ($p<0.0001$) and absolute hepatic excretory rate ($p<0.005$), the very processes that we had previously shown to be impaired in cholestatic diseases (Figure 6). Patients with early stage PBC had a greater improvement than those with late stage disease. It should be remembered that improvement in ^{75}SeHCAT excretion does not prove that excretion of other species of bile acids also improves. From our previous studies[34], it is likely that it mirrors improvement in taurocholate excretion. To our knowledge, comparisons between ^{75}SeHCAT and endogenous hydrophobic bile acids (e.g. chenodeoxycholic acid and deoxycholic acid have not been performed).

PLASMA DISAPPEARANCE MEASUREMENTS

Hepatic uptake and excretion of bile acids can also be assessed indirectly by measuring initial (K_1) and late (K_2) plasma disappearance of ^{75}SeHCAT[36]. These

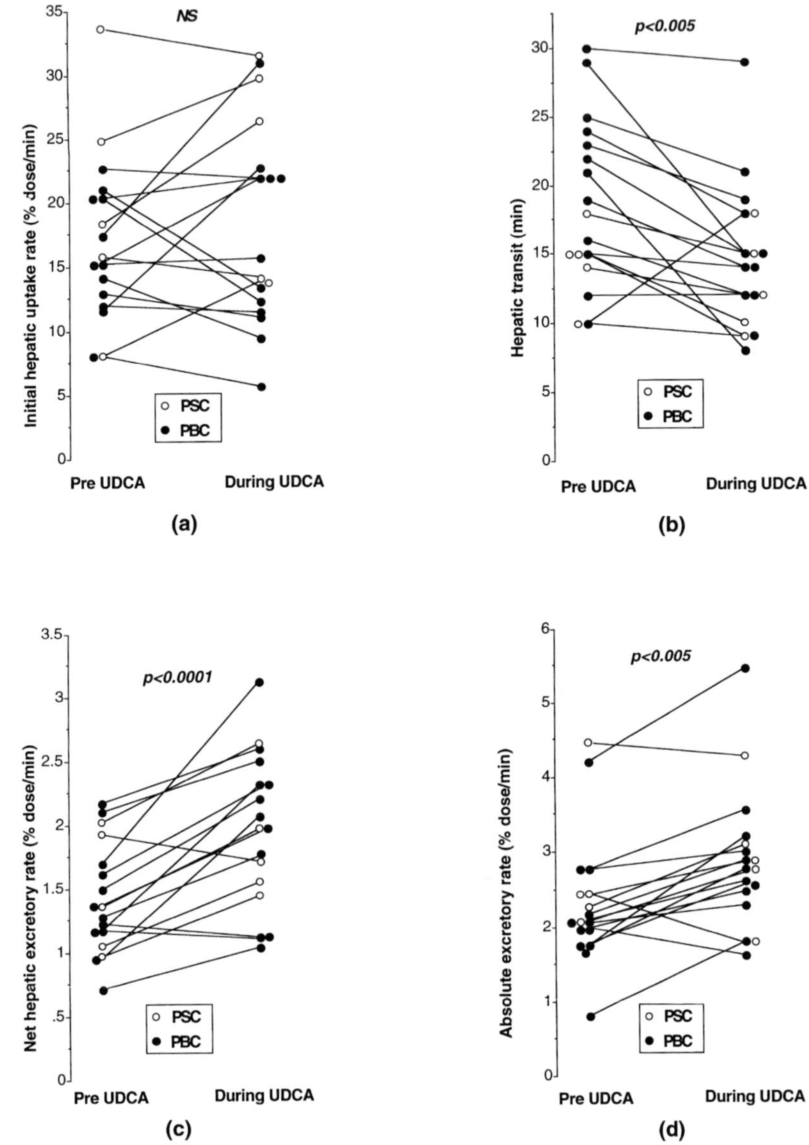

Fig. 6 Effect of UDCA therapy in patients with cholestasis (12 PBC and 5 PSC patients) on: (a) initial hepatic uptake; (b) hepatic transit time; (c) net excretory rate; and (d) absolute excretory rate. The fact that UDCA improves hepatic transit and excretion of bile acids, without affecting uptake, suggests that it reduces intrahepatic bile acid retention (reproduced from reference 35 with permission)

measurements correlate well with the direct scintigraphic measurements of hepatic uptake and excretion. Plasma disappearance by serial blood sampling is easier to perform and does not require the prolonged and continuous use of a

γ-camera. We have also investigated the use another γ-labelled isotope, ^{99m}TcHIDA, to investigate hepatic excretory kinetics by plasma disappearance measurements. This isotope has already been widely used for imaging the hepatobiliary system and for assessing hepatic liver transport function[37,38]. Although less efficiently and specifically handled compared to ^{75}SeHCAT, ^{99m}TcHIDA can also be used to assess hepatic uptake and excretory function and assess the effect of treatment. We have assessed the effect of UDCA on plasma disappearance measurements of ^{99m}TcHIDA in 20 PBC patients studied in a double-blind placebo controlled trial[39]. Improvements in K_2 were detected in PBC patients receiving UDCA but not in those receiving placebo. No improvement in K_1 was detected on either UDCA or placebo.

CONCLUSIONS

Measurement of hepatic uptake and excretion of ^{75}SeHCAT, provides an example of a quantitative and direct test of a dynamic liver function that is both sensitive and specific. Using this test, patients with PBC and PSC are shown to have abnormal hepatic bile acid excretion in the presence of normal hepatic bile acid uptake, thereby confirming intrahepatic bile acid retention at an early stage of the disease. Treatment with UDCA improves hepatic bile acid excretion. Reduction in endogenous hydrophobic bile acid retention may be an important mechanism of action of UDCA in cholestatic liver diseases. Analysis of hepatic bile acid excretion provides an interesting physiological tool for assessing the effects of treatment in these diseases.

References

1. Hofmann AF, Popper H. Ursodeoxycholic acid for primary biliary cirrhosis. Lancet. 1987;398–9.
2. de Caestecker JS, Jazrawi RP, Petroni ML, Northfield TC. Ursodeoxycholic acid in chronic liver disease. Gut. 1991;32:1061–5.
3. Lim AG, Jazrawi RP, Northfield TC. The ursodeoxycholic acid story in primary biliary cirrhosis. Gut. 1995;37:301–4.
4. Poupon RE, Chretien Y, Poupon R, Paumgartner G. Serum bile acids in primary biliary cirrhosis: Effect of ursodeoxycholic acid. Hepatology. 1993;17:599–604.
5. Mazzella G, Parini P, Bazzoli F *et al.* Ursodeoxycholic administration on bile acid metabolism in patients with early stages of primary biliary cirrhosis. Dig Dis Sci. 1993;38:896–902.
6. Beuers U, Spengler U, Zwiebel FM, Pauletzki J, Fischer S, Paumgartner G. Effect of ursodeoxycholic acid on the kinetics of the major hydrophobic bile acids in health and in chronic cholestatic liver disease. Hepatology. 1992;15:603–8.
7. Poupon RE, Poupon R, Balkau B, the UDCA-PBC Study Group. Ursodiol for the longterm treatment of primary biliary cirrhosis. N Engl J Med. 1994;330:1342–7.
8. Poupon RE, Balkau B, Eschwege E, Poupon R, and the UDCA study group. A multicentre double blind trial of ursodiol for the treatment of primary biliary cirrhosis. N Engl J Med. 1991;234:1548–54.
9. Lindor KD, Dixoe ER, BAldus WP *et al.* Ursodeoxycholic acid in the treatment of primary biliary cirrhosis. Gastroenterology. 1994;106:1284–94.
10. Heathcote EJ, Cauch-Dudek K, Walker V *et al.* The Canadian multicentre double blind randomised controlled trial of ursodeoxycholic acid in primary biliary cirrhosis. Hepatology. 1994;19:1149–56.
11. Simko V, Michael S, Prego V. Ursodeoxycholic therapy in chronic liver disease: A meta analysis in primary biliary cirrhosis and in chronic hepatitis. Am J Gastroenterol. 1994;89:392–8.

12. Heathcote EJ, Lindor KD, Poupon R *et al.* Combined analysis of French, American and Canadian randomised controlled trials of ursodeoxycholic acid therapy in primary biliary cirrhosis. Gastroenterology. 1995;108:A1082.
13. Poupon R, Chretien Y, Ballet F, Calmus Y, Darnis F. Is ursodeoxycholic acid an effective treatment in primary biliary cirrhosis. Lancet. 1987;i:834–6.
14. Lotterer E, Stiehl A, Raedsch R, Foelsch UR, Bricher R. Ursodeoxycholic acid in primary biliary cirrhosis: No evidence for toxicity in the stages I to III. J Hepatol. 1990;10:284–90.
15. Huet PM, Willems B, Huet J, Poupon R. Effects of ursodeoxycholic acid on hepatic function and portal hypertention in primary biliary cirrhosis. In: *Proceedings of the VIIth International Bile Acid Meeting*. Basel, Switzerland: Falk Symposium No. 68, 1992:118.
16. Lim AG, Jazrawi RP, Ahmed HA *et al.* Soluble intracellular adhesion molecule-1 in primary biliary cirrhosis: Relationship with disease stage, immune activity and cholestasis. Hepatology. 1994;20:882–8.
17. Lim AG, Jazrawi RP, Levy JH, Douds AC, Maxwell JD, Northfield TC. Soluble E-selection and vascular cell adhesion molecule in primary biliary cirrhosis. J Hepatol. 1995;22:416–22.
18. Lim AG, Wolfhagen FHJ, Verma A *et al.* Combination of ursodeoxycholic acid and immunosuppressive therapy for the treatment of primary biliary cirrhosis. Gut. 1995;37 (Suppl 2):T106.
19. Floreani A, Zappala F, Mazzetto M, Naccarato R, Plebani M, Charamonte M. Different responses to ursodeoxycholic acid (UDCA) in primary biliary cirrhosis according to severity of disease. Dig Dis Sci. 1994;39:9–14.
20. Osterlng C, Aksu T, Somasundaram, R, Stolzel U, Reicken EO, Schuppan D. Serum markers of fibrogenesis and fibrolysis suggest an antifibrotic effect of ursodeoxycholic acid in PBC stage I-IV. International Falk Workshop: Surrogate Markers to Assess Efficacy of Treatment in Chronic Liver Disease. 1995:28.
21. Verma A, Lim AG, Jazrawi RP, Ahmed HA, Northfield TC. Effect of ursodeoxycholic acid on serum markers of fibrosis in primary biliary cirrhosis. Gut. 1995;36 (Suppl 1):A30.
22. Jazrawi RP, Ferraris R, Northfield TC. ^{75}SeHCAT: An overview of its physiological properties and clinical value. In: Northfield TC, Jazrawi RP, Zentler-Munro PL, editors. Bile acids in health and disease. Lancaster: Kluwer Academic, 1988:277–89.
23. Jazrawi RP, Lanzini A, Britten A, Meller ST, Northfield TC. Dynamics of gallbladder functions and of the enterohepatic circulation studied by a γ-labelled bile acid. Clin Sci. 1984;66:10P.
24. Van Berg Henegouwen GP, Hofmann AF. Nocturnal gallbladder storage and emptying in gallstone patients and healthy subjects. Gastroenterology. 1978;75:879–89.
25. Soundy RG, Simpson JD, McL Ross, Merrick MV. Absorbed dose to man from the Se-75-labelled bile salt SeHCAT. J Nucl Med. 1982;23:157–61.
26. Delhez H, Van den Berg JWO, Van Blankenstein M, Meerwald JH. New method for the determination of bile acid turnover using ^{75}Se-homocholic acid taurine. Eur J Nucl Med. 1982;7:269–71.
27. Jazrawi RP, Bridges C, Joseph AEA, Northfield TC. Effects of artificial depletion of the bile acid pool in man. Gut. 1986;27:771–7.
28. Jazrawi RP, Ferraris R, Bridges C, Northfield TC. Kinetics for the synthetic bile acid 75seleno-homocholic acid-taurine in humans: Comparison with [14C] taurocholate. Gastroenterology. 1988;95:164–9.
29. Linstedt S. The turnover of bile acid in man. Acta Physiol Scand. 1957;40:1–9.
30. Merrick MV, Eastwood MA, Anderson JR, Ross J. Enterohepatic circulation in man of a gamma-emitting bile acid conjugate, 23-selena-25-homocholic acid taurine (SeHCAT). J Nucl Med. 1982;23:126–30.
31. Boyd GS, Merrick MV, Monks R, Thomas IL. Se-75-labelled bile acid analogues, new radiopharmaceuticals for investigation. J Nucl Med. 1981;22:720–5.
32. Galatola G, Jazrawi RP, Bridges C, Joseph AEA, Northfield TC. Direct measurement of first pass ileal clearance of a bile acid in humans. Gastroenterology. 1991;100:1100–5.
33. Ferraris R, Jazrawi RP, Bridges C, Northfield TC. Use of a gamma labelled bile acid (^{75}SeHCAT) as a test of ileal function: Methods of improving accuracy. Gastroenterology. 1986;90:1129–36.
34. Galatola G, Jazrawi RP, Bridges C, Joseph AEA, Northfield TC. Hepatic handling of a synthetic γ-labelled bile acid (^{75}SeHCAT). Gastroenterology. 1988;94:771–8
35. Jazrawi RP, de Caestecker JS, Goggin PM *et al.* Kinetics of hepatic bile acid handling in cholestatic liver disease: Effect of ursodeoxycholic acid. Gastroenterology. 1994;106:134–42.

36. de Caestecker JS, Jazrawi RP, Nisbett JA *et al.* Direct assessment of the mechanism for a raised serum bile acid level in chronic liver disease. Eur J Gastroenterol Hepatol. 1995;7:955–61.
37. Gelius L, Skretting A, Aas M. A mathematical model for liver uptake and excretion of 99mTc diethyl IDA. Eur J Nucl Med. 1981;6:139–42.
38. Erjavec M, Pahor S, Poreko DB, Snajder J. Estimation of 99mTc-Diethyl-IDA liver clearance. Eur J Nucl Med. 1982;7:216–21.
39. Lim AG, Jazrawi RP, Maxwel lJD, Northfield TC. Ursodeoxycholic acid improves hepatic excretion in primary biliary cirrhosis. Gut. 1994;35:S11.

19
Surrogate markers to assess efficacy of treatment in viral hepatitis

L. PAGLIARO, M. GIUNTA, C. LINEA, A. CRAXÌ, P. ALMASIO, C. CAMMÀ, V. DI MARCO, S. MAGRIN, A. VACCARO, P. FUSCHI and O. LO IACONO

'TRUE' ENDPOINTS AND 'SURROGATE' ENDPOINTS (OR MARKERS)

Whereas 'true' endpoints of therapeutic efficacy measure a *clinical* benefit (e.g. survival, quality of life, cure of the disease), 'surrogate' endpoints (or markers) actually measure a therapeutic modification of the disease process. Requirements of a surrogate marker are a biological rationale and a sufficient correlation with the true endpoint of interest[1,2].

Surrogate markers are often used as substitutes for true endpoints in randomized clinical trials (RCTs) because they are easier to measure and occur earlier, leading to a reduction of the sample size needed and of the duration of study. Some examples are reported in Table 1[2–4].

Table 1 Surrogate and true endpoints in randomized clinical trials

Disease	*Treatment*	*'True' endpoints*	*Surrogate markers*
Arterial hypertension[2]	Antihypertensives	Prevention of stroke	Blood pressure
Myocardial infarction[2]	Thrombolysis	Survival	Coronary artery patency
Solid tumours[3]	Chemotherapy	Survival	Tumour size
Wilms' tumour[3]	Nephrectomy[1]	Cure	2-yr-survival
Glaucoma[4]	Several drugs	Prevention of blindness	Intraocular pressure

As reported in the table, 'cure' was adopted as the true endpoint of nephrectomy in children's Wilms' tumour, whereas survival during a limited follow-up was used as a surrogate marker.

'Cure' has been the true endpoint in many recent trials of different therapeutic regimens in pulmonary tuberculosis, with sputum conversion, relapse rate and often compliance and adverse reactions used as surrogate markers[5–7].

This is of interest for our topic, since pulmonary tuberculosis has some resemblance with chronic hepatitis C such as infectious origin, strong tendency to chronic course and low mortality.

'TRUE' ENDPOINTS AND SURROGATE MARKERS OF ALPHA-INTERFERON THERAPY FOR CHRONIC HEPATITIS C

We chose to focus this chapter on surrogate markers of alpha interferon (IFN) therapy in chronic hepatitis C because:

- Hepatitis C currently causes cirrhosis and hepatocellular carcinoma (HCC) much more frequently than does hepatitis B in many Western countries[8–10].
- IFN is at present the only approved therapy for the disease throughout the world.

Prevention of death from cirrhosis or HCC would be the most appropriate true endpoint of RCTs of IFN (or other treatments available in the future) for hepatitis C. However, this endpoint is impractical for several reasons:

- The course of HCV-related chronic liver disease is exceedingly prolonged and indolent, with a mortality ranging between 2 and 10% in patients with chronic hepatitis followed for 10 to 18 years. Moreover, the number of deaths unrelated to liver disease in the published studies was higher than liver-related mortality, possibly confounding the evaluation of results (Table 2). Therefore a very large sample size and an extended duration of RCTs would be required.
- An RCT comparing treated patients and untreated controls to assess the efficacy of IFN on disease-related mortality would be unrealistic and unethical.
- Prevention of mortality would be an endpoint unsuitable for decision making in the individual patient during the course of disease.

Cure of chronic hepatitis C, defined as the stable disappearance of both necroinflammatory processes in the liver and markers of HCV infection is a preferable true endpoint of therapeutic efficacy. It can be assessed within a reasonable period of time and can lead the therapeutic strategy in the individual patient.

We aim to identify the indicators of 'cure'; the time-point during or after IFN therapy at which a sufficiently high probability of cure or failure can be established; and the predictors of cure during and shortly after therapy.

Methods

We used data from the relevant literature and a database of two RCTs performed in our unit. By Medline and manual search we located studies (mostly RCTs) in

Table 2 Mortality in hepatitis C

			% Deaths		*Hepatitis at onset of follow-up*	
Study	*No. of pts*	*Mean follow-up (yrs)*	*Liver specific*	*All causes*	*Acute/ chronic*	*Type of hepatitis*
The Copenhagen HA Programme[11]	142	4.8	1.4	7.7	Acute	PTH
Mattson *et al.*[12]	37	2.8	None	None	Chronic	PTH
Mattson *et al.*[13]	92	~5	None	4.3	Chronic	PTH + community
Di Bisceglie *et al.*[14]	33	9.7	1.6	27.2	Chronic	PTH
Wejstal *et al.*[15]	127	6.3	0.7	3.1	Chronic	PTH + community
Seeff *et al.*[16]	568	18	3.3	47.1	Acute	PTH
Tremolada *et al.*[17]	104	7.5	4.8	10.5	Chronic	PTH
Koretz *et al.*[18]	55	16	3.6	14	Chronic	PTH
Sanchez-Tapias[19]	305	9.5	7	n.r.	Chronic	PTH + community

PTH, post-transfusion hepatitis; n.r., not reported

which IFN-treated patients with chronic hepatitis C were monitored during therapy and followed long-term after IFN cessation with serial determinations of ALT and HCV-RNA by polymerase chain reaction (PCR).

Data dealing with the same issues were also abstracted from two RCTs now concluded at our unit[20], in which a total of 426 patients with chronic hepatitis C (41% with cirrhosis, 81% from HCV genotype 1b) were enrolled. Patients were treated with 10 to 5 MU of lymphoblastoid (first trial) or recombinant (second trial) IFN for 6 or 12 months, and then followed long-term.

IDENTIFICATION OF CURE AS THE TRUE ENDPOINT: ALT AND HCV-RNA FOR 1 YEAR AFTER IFN CESSATION

From the pool of studies located in the literature we identified 6 studies in which patients with stable normal ALT and negative HCV-RNA at the end of therapy (primary responders) were followed for more than 12 months. The same type of data were drawn from our RCTs.

As shown in Table 3, only one (or perhaps 2) among 179 patients maintaining normal ALT and negative HCV-RNA for 1-year after IFN cessation, relapsed during subsequent follow-up, ranging between 12 and 60 months. No relapses were reported between the sixth and the twelfth month of follow-up in the five studies where data were available.

Therefore, using a conservative approach to these data, we suggest that the combination of stable normal ALT and negative HCV-RNA 12 months after IFN cessation can be assumed as 'cure' of chronic hepatitis C in almost all patients. However, since later relapses can still occur, prolonged ALT monitoring would be warranted in these subjects.

Two other findings are of interest:

1. Among patients with stable normal ALT without relapses for 12 months after the end of IFN, the majority are HCV-RNA negative at the end of therapy (74% and 84% in the two larger studies)[25,26].
2. Although some patients with normal ALT and positive HCV-RNA at 12 months exhibit later relapses[25], others maintain normal ALT over 3–4 years[22,25,26].

Table 3 Long-term course of patients with stable normal ALT and negative serum HCV-RNA for 1 year after the end of IFN (6 studies)

Study	*Pts with normal ALT and negative HCV-RNA at 6 and 12 months*	*Subsequent mean follow-up (mo)*	*Late relapses*
Shindo *et al.*[21]	6	24–60	None
Saracco *et al.*[22]	9[a]	34	One
Camps *et al.*[23]	14	28	None
Reichard *et al.*[24]	14	12	One
Alberti[25]	80	22	None
Lo Iacono *et al.*[26]	56	12	None

[a]Data at 6 months not available

Identification of predictors of cure as surrogate markers: ALT and HCV-RNA during and at the end of IFN therapy

Prediction of 'cure' (persistently normal ALT and negative HCV-RNA for 12 months after IFN cessation) is of interest for decision making. Therefore we attempted to identify predictors in studies in which patients were observed for at least 12 months after the end of therapy.

Figure 1 shows the rates of 1-year complete response (cure) after IFN cessation in our RCTs, as related to the results of ALT determinations during the treatment.

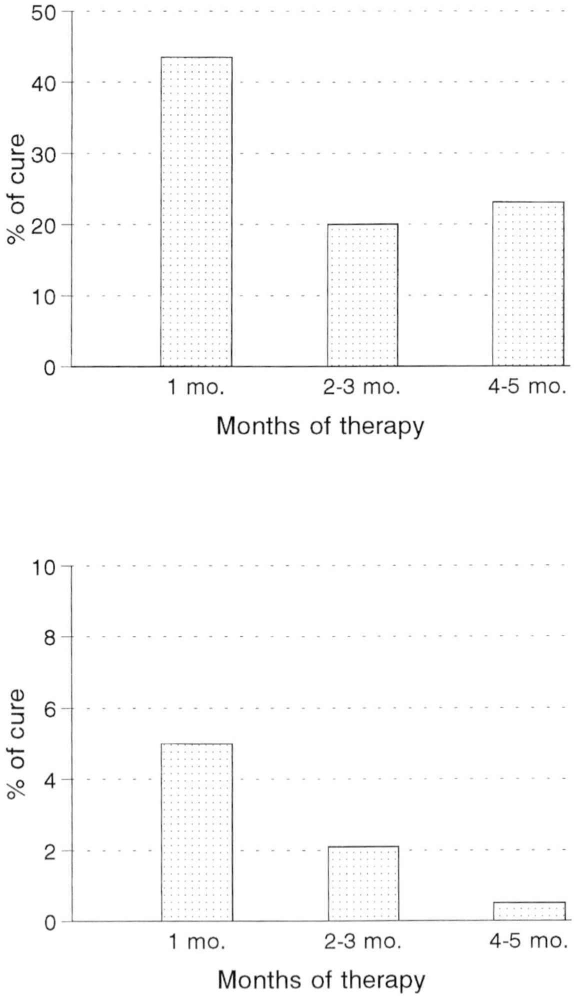

Fig. 1 Probability of 'cure' (i.e. normal ALT and negative serum HCV-RNA for 12 months after IFN cessation) as related to the time of ALT normalization or to persistently abnormal ALT during therapy[35]

As shown in the upper panel, patients with normal ALT during the first month of IFN have a higher probability of cure than those with later ALT normalization. However, even among patients with early primary response, the cure rate does not exceed 43%. Of interest is the finding (lower panel) that the probability of cure is very low in patients with abnormal ALT after 1, 3 or 5 months of IFN, declining from 5% after 1 month of 2.8% and 0.5% after 3 and 5 months, respectively.

Table 4 shows the low rate of primary response in patients in which ALT has not normalized within 3 months of IFN, as reported in 23 RCTs (21 located in the meta-analysis of Bardelli *et al.* and re-evaluated)[27–29]: as shown in the table, only 3% of 521 patients with still abnormal ALT at 3 months achieved a primary response, independently of the total duration of therapy.

Since patients achieving long-term cure are a fraction of primary responders, these data provide sufficient evidence that the probability of cure is exceedingly low if ALT is still abnormal after 3 months of IFN.

Table 5 shows that negative serum HCV-RNA during IFN therapy has a predictive value for 'cure' closely similar to normal ALT: only 43% of patients with negative HCV-RNA after 3 months of IFN will become long-term responders. On the other hand, a positive HCV-RNA at 3 months is predictive of low probability of cure even in the presence of normal ALT (9.5%). Early HCV-RNA disappearance in responders has also been reported by Brouwer *et al.* in abstract form[31] with more than 95% of the total HCV-RNA response occurring within 1 month.

ALT and HCV-RNA are poorly predictive of long-term response even at IFN cessation: 6- or 12-month sustained response rates are about 50% in patients with ALT primary response (Figure 2) or with negative HCV-RNA (Figure 3, upper panel)[29,32–35] at that time. On the other hand, very few patients with abnormal ALT (7 out of 186 patients in our RCTs) or positive HCV-RNA (Figure 3, lower panel)[29,33,35] escape relapse in the first few months after IFN cessation.

THE ROLE OF HISTOLOGY TO SUPPORT OR PREDICT CURE

Histological examination of liver biopsy specimens is a time-honoured and important tool in hepatology. Hence, it is not surprising that many studies report

Table 5 ALT and serum HCV-RNA at the third month of IFN therapy for prediction of 'cure'[a] in chronic hepatitis C (106 pts)

	% Cure
Patients with abnormal ALT	None
Patients with normal ALT:	
– and HCV-RNA positive	9.5
– and HCV-RNA negative	43.7

[a]Cure: normal ALT and serum HCV-RNA negative for 6 months after treatment (from reference 30)

Table 4 Proportion of patients with primary response who had abnormal ALT after 3 months of IFN

3-mo-abnormal ALT[a] / *Primary response* %	*No. of RCTs*	*3-mo-abnormal ALT*[a] / *Primary response* (*Total no. of pts in the RCTs*)	*No. of RCTs with duration of therapy* ≤*6 mo*/≥*6 mo*
None	14	None/302	9/5
None to 5%	1	2/185	None/1
Between 5 and 15%	6	9/77	4/2
Between 15 and 35%	2	4/17	1/1
			Total: 3-mo-abnormal ALT[a] / Primary response: 15/521 (3.2%)

[a] 3-mo-abnormal ALT / Primary response = Pts with abnormal ALT after 3 months of IFN / Pts with primary response at the end of IFN therapy

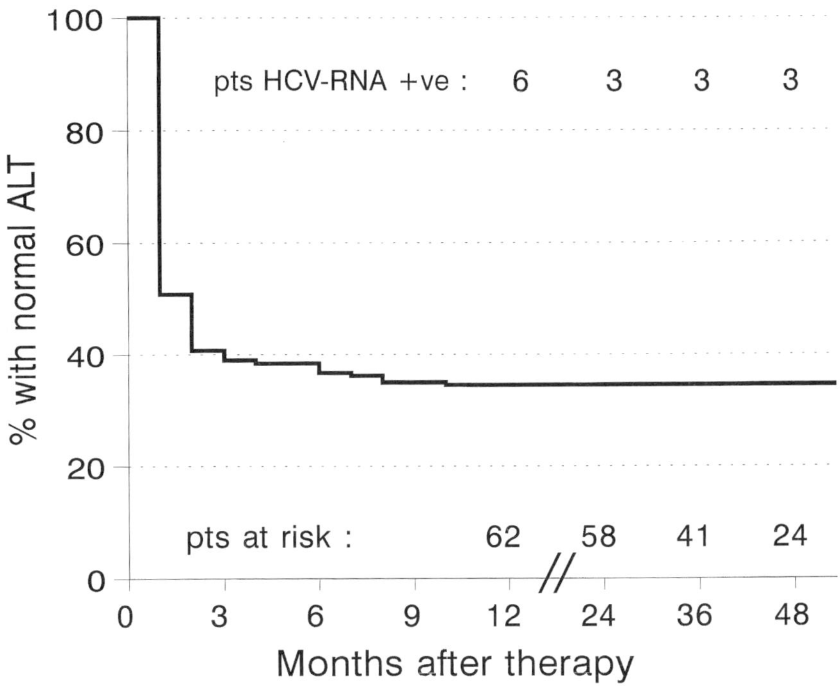

Fig. 2 Incidence of ALT relapses after IFN cessation in two RCTs[35,36]

a comparative assessement of liver histological findings in biopsies taken before and after IFN therapy. However, the histological approach to the evaluation of IFN response in chronic hepatitis C has several important limitations and sources of bias:

- The attempt to perform a semi-quantitative assessment of histological lesions undergoes a sizeable inter-observer variation, particularly by non-specialized pathologists.
- The histological activity index (HAI) by Knodell's method or its modifications is measured on an ordinal scale with non-constant intervals, possibly leading to bias in the cumulative or comparative assessment of data.
- The histological picture of chronic hepatitis C is mild to moderate in most cases; as a result, the relatively small changes induced by IFN can be difficult to assess with precision, increasing the inter-observer variation.
- The biopsy specimen reflects just one point in a long-term process evolving at a variable speed, but liver biopsy is an invasive procedure that cannot be repeated again and again.

Taking these limitations into account, we regard the IFN-induced histological changes reported here as an approximate (although important) indication of treatment effect; they are not a precise quantitative estimate.

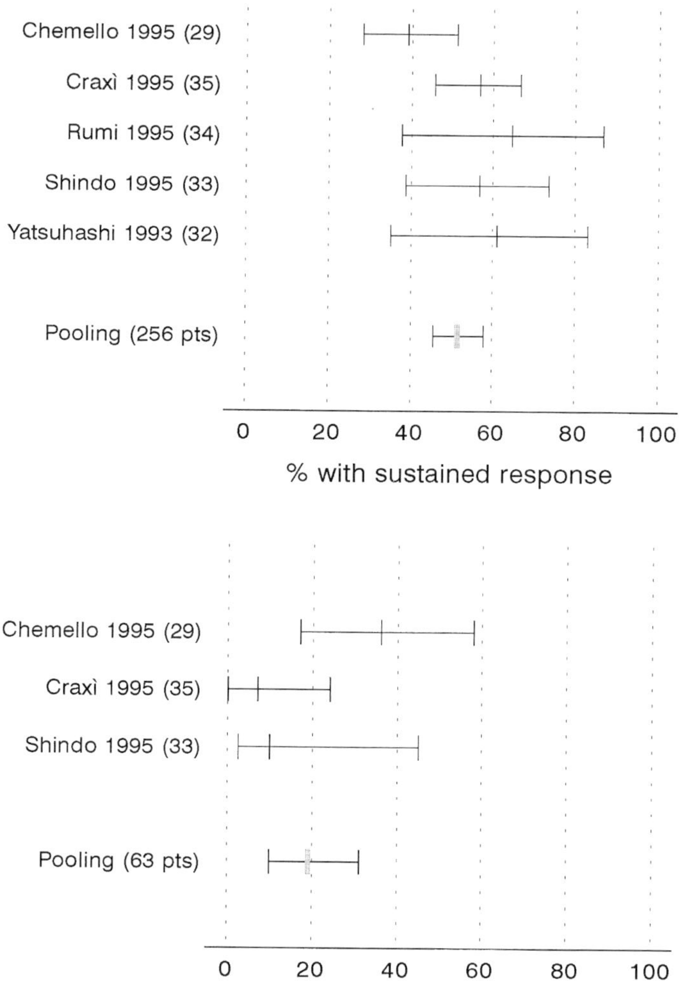

Fig. 3 Probability of 6 or 12 months long-term ALT response as related to HCV-RNA status at IFN cessation (only studies including 10 or more patients are reported)

Histological changes in long-term IFN responders or relapsers

Performing a liver biopsy after a long-term complete IFN response or in relapsers is not easy for patients to accept and is questionable as a current practice.

Data on this issue are therefore limited. Shindo *et al.*[33], found that HAI decreased from the initial score of 9.3 to 2.2 in 22 patients with sustained ALT and virological response 1 year after IFN cessation. The corresponding findings of Craxi *et al.*[35] were 10.8 and 4.3; negligible changes were found in relapsers (from 9.8 to 8.9). Chemello *et al.*[29] found histological improvement in 72% of patients with normal ALT for 6–12 months after IFN cessation (81% in those with normal ALT and negative HCV-RNA); the histological picture improved in 35% of relapsers. However, post-treatment biopsies were normal or showed minimal changes in only 48% of the long-term responders, suggesting that a longer period of time is required for the complete regression of necro-inflammatory changes in many patients achieving 'cure'. This is confirmed by the limited data in patients with more prolonged ALT and HCV-RNA response: spotty and piecemeal necrosis disappeared after 2 years in 14 patients[24]; and a normal histological picture was found after 3 years in 4 patients[22].

Histological changes at the end of therapy

The comparative examination of liver biopsies taken before and at the end of IFN has been used in several RCTs to support the reduction of the necroinflammatory process suggested by the ALT response.

1. The comparison between untreated controls and IFN-treated patients (aggregating together ALT responders and non-responders) is shown in Tables 6 and 7. Table 6 shows changes of HAI score in 10 RCTs, usually assessed by Knodell's method or its modifications. A reduction was found in treated groups in all RCTs, ranging between 45% and 18% of the initial value (median: 28%); the reduction was greater in necroinflammation than in fibrosis, which was often not affected at all. No or very few changes occurred in controls. Table 7 shows the percentages of treated and control patients with an improved histological picture in 7 RCTs. The median

Table 6 HAI score before and at the end of IFN therapy in 10 RCTs comparing treated patients and untreated controls

		Mean HAI score					
		Treated patients			*Controls*		
Study	*No. of pts*	*Basal (B)*	*Final (F)*	*% Difference (F – B)*	*Basal (B)*	*Final (F)*	*% Difference (F – B)*
Di Bisceglie *et al.*[37]	41	11.8	9.7	–17.8	12.7	12.4	–2.3
Gomez-Rubio *et al.*[38]	30	11.2	8.3	–25.9	9.1	8.3	–8.8
Saracco *et al.*[22]	90	9.1	7.3	–19.8	8.1	8.4	+3.7
Manabe *et al.*[39]	90	10.31	7.1	–31.1	10.2	9.0	–11.7
Omata *et al.*[40]	49	9.5	7.0	–26.3	8.5	8.5	0
Marcellin *et al.*[41]	60	8.9	5.9	–33.7	8.7	7.2	–17.2
Schvarcz *et al.*[42]	31	3.4	2.3	–32.3	4.3	3.7	–13.9
Camps *et al.*[23]	72	10.86	6.8	–37.4	9.25	9.53	+3.0
De Alava *et al.*[43]	89	10.82	8.14	–24.7	10.14	9.7	–4.3
Saez-Royuela *et al.*[44]	30	9.8	5.7	–41.8	13.3	14.4	+8.2

Table 7 Percentage of patients with histological improvement at the end of IFN therapy in 7 RCTs comparing treated patients (≥3MU tiw for ≥4 months) and untreated controls

	% of pts with histological picture improved		
	No. of pts	*Treated patients*	*Controls*
Wejland *et al.*[45]	33	78	50
David *et al.*[46]	90	68	33
Camps *et al.*[23]	72	91	25
Diodati *et al.*[47]	60	28	0
Davis *et al.*[48]	166	52	n.r.
Manabe *et al.*[39]	90	73	?
Castilla *et al.*[49]	40	85	5

n.r., not reported

reduction was 73% in the IFN-treated groups (range from 91% to 28%) and 25% in controls (range from 50% to none).

2. Table 8 shows the comparison between patients with ALT normalization (primary responders), non-responders and partial responders (i.e. those with ALT reduction, usually by 50% or more, not reaching the normal range). The basal HAI score appreciably decreased in responders in 4 studies (median: 32.6% reduction; range from 53 to 24%) reduction. Very few changes were found in non-responders (the largest reduction was 19,6%). A separate evaluation in partial responders was reported only in 2 studies[51,52], showing a reduction of 36% and 27%, respectively.

Overall, these data show that IFN decreases the histological features of necroinflammation in chronic hepatitis C, particularly in patients with ALT normalization. The limited observations available suggest that histological improvement is also associated with partial ALT reduction. This is in agreement with the findings of Poynard *et al.*[53], that showed histological

Table 8 HAI score before and at the end of IFN therapy: comparison between patients with primary ALT response (CR) and non-(NR) or partial-(PR) response in five studies

		Mean HAI score					
		CR			*NR + PR*		
Study	*No. of pts*	*Basal (B)*	*Final (F)*	*% Difference (F – B)*	*Basal (B)*	*Final (F)*	*% Difference (F – B)*
Saracco *et al.*[22]	90	8.9	6.0	–32.5	9.2	8.4	–8.6
Marcellin *et al.*[41]	60	9.8	6.4	–34.7	9.1	8.9	–2.2
Perez *et al.*[50]	73	11.31	7.62	–32.6	11.06	7.06	–36.1[a]
Yamada *et al.*[51]	70	8.9	4.1	–53.9	10.7	7.8	–27.1[a]
					12.0	11.4	–5[b]
Mazzella *et al.*[52]	60	8.58	6.5	–24.2	8.15	6.55	–19.6

[a]Only PR
[b]Only NR

improvement even in patients with 'abnormal' ALT, presumably including some partial responders.

3. Table 9 shows the comparison between long-term responders and relapsers in four studies. The median percentage difference between HAI score at the onset and at the end of IFN was greater in long-term responders (54% decrease; range 55% to 41% decrease) than in relapsers (21% decrease; range 38% to 7% decrease).

Table 9 HAI score before and at the end of IFN therapy: Comparison between future long-term responders (LTR) and relapsers (REL) in five studies

		HAI score (mean ± SD)					
		LTR			*REL*		
Study	*No. of pts*	*Basal (B)*	*Final (F)*	*% Difference (F – B)*	*Basal (B)*	*Final (F)*	*% Difference (F – B)*
Saracco *et al.*[22]	90	9.2	4.1	–55.4	8.8	8.2	–6.8
Camps *et al.*[23]	72	11.8	5.6	–52.5	8.87	6.12	–31.0
De Alava *et al.*[43]	89	11.2	6.62	–41.1	10.21	8.7	–14.8
Shindo *et al.*[33]	47	9.3	4.2	–54.8	9.2	5.7	–38.0

DISCUSSION

The mortality of untreated patients with autoimmune chronic active hepatitis was as high as 28 to 55% during the first 2–6 years after the diagnosis. Reduction of mortality was therefore easily evaluated as the true endpoint in the RCTs of immunosuppressive treatments[54–56].

In chronic hepatitis C, reduction of mortality would be a non-realistic endpoint of treatment, since very few deaths occur for 10–20 years after diagnosis (Table 2). Therefore, the first aim of the present study was the identification of an assessable and clinically significant endpoint of IFN therapy. The choice of stable normality of ALT associated with negative HCV-RNA for 1 year after the end of therapy has a biological rationale and an observational justification as an indicator of 'cure'.

In fact, although several studies have found necroinflammation at liver histology despite normal ALT in HCV-RNA *positive* patients[57,58], subjects with normal ALT and *negative* HCV-RNA after IFN achieve regression of necroinflammation in the long term[22,24].

Moreover, although HCV might undergo late reactivation in patients without circulating HCV-RNA, the long-term negativity of this marker for 2–6 years is encouraging.

Predictors of 'cure' or failure of 'cure' can be seen as 'surrogate markers' of IFN efficacy. We found that abnormal ALT, positive HCV-RNA, or their combination, after 3 months of IFN, are predictive of the failure of 'cure', independent of the duration of treatment (Table 4). This finding is not in conflict with some RCTs[29,53,59] showing that the sustained response rate after 12 or 18 months is higher than after 6 months of IFN: the length of therapy might stabilize the early IFN response in some patients, not increase the primary response rate. If so, the identification of markers predictive of the long-term response or relapse in such patients would be of value.

Almost none of the patients with increased ALT and positive HCV-RNA (or, perhaps with positive HCV-RNA and normal ALT) at the third month of IFN therapy or at cessation of therapy will achieve 'cure'. This finding can be used for decision making: patients with increased ALT and perhaps also those with normal ALT and positive HCV-RNA after 3 months of IFN should be switched to a different treatment (or to a different IFN regimen, or to a combination of drugs). On the contrary, about half of the patients with normal ALT and/or negative HCV-RNA will relapse, and half will achieve 'cure'. Markers predictive of the long-term disease course after IFN cessation in these patients are not available nowadays, although they would be of help for therapeutic strategy.

The consistent improvement of HAI score in liver biopsies taken at the end of therapy in responders is important because it confirms the evidence of efficacy of IFN suggested by ALT normalization. Even more important to support the concept of 'cure' of chronic hepatitis C is the complete or nearly complete regression of active histological lesions in most patients with long-term ALT and HCV-RNA response. However, methodological problems and the limited number of biopsies that can be performed in each patient do not allow the use of histology in assessment of IFN response and in decision making.

SUMMARY

1. Almost all patients with normal ALT and negative serum HCV-RNA for 1 year after IFN cessation maintain the long-term response for several years. Therefore, one-year stable normal ALT and negative HCV-RNA can be assumed as an endpoint, suggesting 'cure' of IFN-treated chronic hepatitis C.
2. The complete or nearly complete regression of histological necro-inflammatory lesions in 2–3 year long-term responders confirms the 'cure' and supports the evidence given by ALT normalization.
3. Abnormal ALT or positive HCV-RNA at the third month of IFN or at the end of therapy predict non-response or relapse, and suggest a therapeutic modification. On the other hand, normality of either marker is not predictive of cure, since about 50% of patients with primary response experience relapse. Markers predictive of long-term response or relapse in these patients would help in planning therapeutic strategies.

Acknowledgements

The Authors are indebted to Mrs Clara Profeta and Mr Antonio Lino for their invaluable secretarial assistance. This work was supported in part by a grant of the Ministero dell'Universita e della Ricerca Scientifica e Tecnologica of Italy.

References

1. Herson J. The use of surrogate endpoints in clinical trials (an introduction to series of four papers). Stat Med. 1989;8:403–4.

2. Wittes J, Lakatos E, Probstfield J. Surrogate endpoints in clinical trials: Cardiovascular disease. Stat Med. 1989;8:415–25.
3. Ellenberg S, Hamilton JM. Surrogate endpoints in clinical trials: Cancer. Stat Med. 1989;8:405–13.
4. Hillis A, Seigel D. Surrogate endpoints in clinical trials: Ophtalmologic disorders. Stat Med. 1989;8:427–30.
5. Zierski M, Bek E, Long MW, Snider DE Jr. Short course (6 month) cooperative tuberculosis study in Poland: Results 18 months after completion of treatment. Am Rev Respir Dis. 1980;122:879–89.
6. Hong Kong Chest Service/British Medical Research Council. Five-year follow-up of a controlled trial of five 6-month regiments of chemotherapy for pulmonary tuberculosis. Am Rev Respir Dis. 1987;136:1339–42.
7. Combs DL, O'Brien RJ, Geiter L. USPHS tuberculosis short-course chemotherapy trial 21: Effectiveness, toxicity and acceptability. The report of final results. Ann Intern Med. 1990;112:397–406.
8. De Bac C, Stroffolini T, Gaeta GB, Taliani G, Giusti G. Pathogenic factors in cirrhosis with and without hepatocellular carcinoma: A multicenter Italian study. Hepatology. 1994;20:1225–30.
9. Roudot-Thoraval F, Bastie A, Pawlotsky JM, Dhumeaux D and the Study Group of the Prevalence and the Epidemiology of Hepatitis C. Risk factors for cirrhosis with chronic hepatitis C J Hepatol. 1995;23 (Suppl 1):101 (abstract).
10. Roudot-Thoraval F, Bastie A, Pawlotsky JM, Dhumeaux D and the Study Group of the Prevalence and the Epidemiology of Hepatitis C. Which factors influence the occurrence of hepatocellular carcinoma in patients with chronic hepatitis C. J Hepatol. 1995;23 (Suppl 1):110 (abstract).
11. The Copenhagen Hepatitis Acuta Programme. Mortality after acute hepatitis type A,B and non-A non-B in 981 patients followed up to 10 years. Scand J Gastroenterol. 1982;17:193–8.
12. Mattsson L, Weiland O, Glaumann H. Long-term follow-up of chronic post-transfusion non-A, non-B hepatitis: Clinical and histological outcome. Liver. 1988;8:184–8.
13. Mattsson L, Weiland O, Glaumann H. Chronic non-A, non-B hepatitis developed after transfusions, illicit self-injections or sporadically. Outcome during long-term follow-up – a comparison. Liver. 1989;9:120–7.
14. Di Bisceglie AM, Goodman ZD, Ishak KG, Hoofnagle JH, Melpolder JJ and Alter HJ. Long-term clinical and histopathological follow-up of chronic posttransfusion hepatitis. Hepatology. 1991;14:969–74.
15. Wejstal R, Hermodsson S, Norkrans G. Long-term follow-up of chronic hepatitis non-A, non-B with special reference to hepatitis C. Liver. 1991;11:143–8.
16. Seeff LB, Buskell-Bales Z, Wright EC *et al.* Long-term mortality after transfusion-associated non-A, non-B hepatitis. N Engl J Med. 1992;327:1906–11.
17. Tremolada F, Casarin C, Alberti A *et al.* Long-term follow-up of non-A, non-B (type C) post-transfusion hepatitis. J Hepatol. 1992;16:273–81.
18. Koretz RL, Abbey H, Coleman E, Gitnick G. Non-A, non-B post-transfusion hepatitis. Looking back in the second decade. Ann Intern Med. 1993;119:110–5.
19. Courtesy of Prof. JM Sanchez-Tapias (unpublished data).
20. Pagliaro L, Craxi A, Camma C *et al.* Interferon for chronic hepatitis C: An analysis of pretreatment clinical predictors of response. Hepatology. 1994;19:820–8.
21. Shindo M, Di Bisceglie AM, Hoofnagle JH. Long-term follow-up of patients with chronic hepatitis C treated with alpha-interferon. Hepatology. 1992;15:1013–6.
22. Saracco G, Rosina F, Abate ML *et al.* Long-term follow-up of patients with chronic hepatitis C treated with different doses of interferon-alpha$_{2b}$. Hepatology. 1993;18:1300–5.
23. Camps J, Castilla A, Ruiz J, Civeira MP, Prieto J. Randomised trial of lymphoblastoid alpha-interferon in chronic hepatitis C. Effects on inflammation, fibrogenesis and viremia. J Hepatol. 1993;17:390–6.
24. Reichard O, Glaumann H, Fryden A *et al.* Two-year biochemical virological and histological follow-up in patients with chronic hepatitis C responding in a sustained fashion to interferon alpha$_{2b}$ treatment. Hepatology. 1995;21:918–22.
25. Courtesy of Prof. A. Alberti (from a paper accepted for publication in Ann Intern Med).
26. Lo Iacono O, Di Marco V, Vaccaro A *et al.* Long-term response to interferon: Effects on viral replication and liver histology. J Hepatol. 1995;23:(Suppl 1) 90 (Abstract).

27. Bardelli F, Messori A, Rampazzo R, Alberti A, Martini N. Effect of recombinant or lymphoblastoid interferon-alpha on alanine aminotransferase in patients with chronic hepatitis C or chronic non-A, non-B hepatitis. Clin Drug Invest. 1995;9:239–54.
28. Attili AF, Natali L, Onori L, Festuccia V, Natali GF. Treatment of type C chronic active hepatitis with interferon-alpha-2a. J Clin Gastroenterol. 1994;19(3):214–6.
29. Chemello L, Bonetti P, Cavalletto L *et al.* Randomized trial comparing three different regimens of alpha-2a-interferon in chronic hepatitis C. Hepatology. 1995;22:700–6.
30. Pol S, Jaffredo F, Nalpas B, Sayada C, Berthelot P, Br!echot C. Undetectable HCV viremia after 3 months of IFN is predictor of long-term response (LTR). J Hepatol. 1995;23:(Suppl 1) 105 (Abstract).
31. Brouwer JT, Nevens F, Kleter GEM *et al.* Efficacy of Interferon dose and factors predictive of sustained response in chronic hepatitis C: Final results of a Benelux multicentre study in 350 patients. J Hepatol. 1995;23:(Suppl 1) 85 (Abstract).
32. Yatsuhashi H, Inoue O, Inokuchi K *et al.* Short and long-term effects of interferon on serum markers of hepatitis C virus replication. J Gastroenterol Hepatol. 1993;8:1–6.
33. Shindo M, Arai K, Yoshihiro S, Okuno T. Hepatic hepatitis C virus RNA as a predictor of long-term response to interferon-therapy. Ann Intern Med. 1995;122:586–91.
34. Rumi MG, Del Ninno E, Parravicini ML *et al.* Long-term titrated recombinant interferon-2a in chronic hepatitis C: randomized controlled trial. J Viral Hepatitis. 1995;2:73–6.
35. Craxi A, Di Marco V, Lo Iacono O *et al.* Transfusion-associated chronic hepatitis C: alpha-n 1 interferon for 6 vs. 12 months. J Hepatol. (accepted for publication).
36. Craxi A, Lo Iacono O, Di Marco V *et al.* Community-acquired chronic hepatitis C in an area of high serotype 1 endemicity: Interferon for 6 or 12 months? Hepatology. 1994;20:155A.
37. Di Bisceglie A, Martin P, Kassianides C *et al.* Recombinant interferon alfa therapy for chronic hepatitis C. A randomized, double-blind, placebo-controlled trial. N Engl J Med. 1989;321:1506–10.
38. Gomez-Rubio M, Porres JC, Castillo I, Quiroga J A, Moreno A, Carreno V. Prolonged treatment (18 months) of chronic hepatitis C with recombinant-interferon in comparison with a control group. J Hepatol. 1990;11:S63–7.
39. Manabe N, Chevallier M, Chossegros P *et al.* Interferon-2b therapy reduces liver fibrosis in chronic non-A, non-B hepatitis: A quantitative histological evaluation. Hepatology. 1993;18:1344–9.
40. Omata M, Ito Y, Yokosuka O *et al.* Randomized, double-blind, placebo-controlled trial of eight-week course of recombinant-interferon for chronic non-A, non-B hepatitis. Dig Dis Sci. 1991:36:1217–22.
41. Marcellin P, Boyer N, Giostra E *et al.* Recombinant human-interferon in patients with chronic non-A, non-B hepatitis: A multicenter randomized controlled trial from France. Hepatology. 1991;13:393–7.
42. Schvarcz R, Glaumann H, Weiland O, Norkrans G, Wejstal R, Fryden A. Histological outcome in interferon alpha-2b treated patients with chronic posttransfusion non-A, non-B hepatitis. Liver. 1991;11:30–8.
43. De Alava E, Camps J, Pardo-Mindan J *et al.* Histological outcome of chronic hepatitis C treated with a 12-month course of lymphoblastoid alfa interferon. Liver. 1993;13:73–9.
44. Saez-Royuela F, Porres JC, Moreno A *et al.* High doses of recombinant-interferon or interferon for chronic hepatitis C: A randomized controlled trial. Hepatology. 1991;13:327–31.
45. Wejland O, Schvarcz R, Wejstal R, Norkrans G, Frydén A. Therapy of chronic post-transfusion non-A, non-B hepatitis with interferon alfa-2b: Swedish experience. J Hepatol. 1990;11:S57–62.
46. David E, Pucci A, Palladin D *et al.* Histologic changes in liver biopsy specimens produced by recombinant interferon-2b therapy for chronic non-A, non-B viral hepatitis. A randomized controlled trial. Am J Clin Pathol. 1992;98:397–401.
47. Diodati G, Bonetti P, Noventa F *et al.* Treatment of chronic hepatitis C with recombinant human interferon-2a: results of a randomized controlled clinical trial. Hepatology. 1994;19:1–5
48. Davis GL, Balart LA, Schiff ER *et al.* Treatment of chronic hepatitis C with recombinant interferon-alfa. A multicenter randomized, controlled trial. N Engl J Med. 1989;321:1501–6.
49. Castilla A, Camps-Bansell J, Civeira MP, Prieto J. Lymphoblastoid-Interferon for chronic hepatitis C: a randomized controlled study. Am J Gastroenterol. 1993;88:233–9.
50. Pérez R, Pravia R, Linares A *et al.* Treatment of chronic hepatitis C with recombinant alfa-2b for nine months. Gut. 1993;(suppl):S136–S138.

51. Yamada G, Takahashi M, Endo H *et al.* Quantitative hepatitis C virus RNA and liver histology in chronic patients treated with interferon alfa. Gut. 1993; (suppl):S133–S134.
52. Mazzella G, Salzetta A, Casanova S *et al.* Treatment of chronic sporadic-type non-A, non-B hepatitis with lymphoblastoid interferon: gamma GT levels predictive for response. Dig Dis Sci. 1994;39:866–70.
53. Poynard T, Bedossa P, Chevallier M *et al.* A comparison of three interferon alfa-2b regimens for the long-term treatment of chronic non-A, non-B hepatitis. N Engl J Med. 1995;332:1457–62.
54. Cook GC, Mulligan R, Sherlock S. Controlled prospective trial of corticosteroid therapy in active chronic hepatitis. Q J Med. 1971;40:159–85.
55. Soloway RD, Summerskill WHJ, Baggenstoss AH, Geall MG, Gitnick GL, Elveback LR, Schoenfield LJ. Clinical, biochemical and histological remission of severe chronic active liver disease: a controlled study of treatments and early prognosis. Gastroenterology. 1972;63:820–33.
56. Murray-Lyon IM, Stern RB, Williams R. Controlled trial of prednisolone and azothioprine in active chronic hepatitis. Lancet. 1973;i:735–7.
57. Alberti A, Morsica G, Chemello L *et al.* Hepatitis C viremia and liver disease in symptom-free individuals with anti-HCV. Lancet. 1992;340:697–8.
58. Shindo M, Arai K, Sokagua Y, Okuno T. The virological and histological states of anti-hepatitis C virus-positive subjects with normal liver biochemical values. Hepatology. 1995;22:418–25.
59. Kasahara A, Hayashi N, Hiramatsu N *et al.* Ability of prolonged interferon treatment to suppress relapse after cessation of therapy in patients with chronic hepatitis C: A multicenter randomized controlled trial. Hepatology. 1995;21:291–7.

20
Surrogate markers in chronic liver disease – poster session

J. SCHÖLMERICH

Treatment of chronic liver disease can have different aims. The optimal result would be to eliminate the cause of disease – this is, however, only rarely possible. Therefore most treatments aim at slowing down progression to cirrhosis and reducing the impact of complications in order to improve survival. In more advanced situations, alleviation of symptoms and even the improvement of conventional markers of liver disease have been the aims of treatment (Table 1).

From this unfortunate scenario currently used markers of treatment success can be obtained. A change in survival has only been found in very few situations, i.e. consequent venaesectio in genetic haemochromatosis[1] or penicillamine in Wilson's disease. There has been greater success for the reduction of the impact of complications such as treatment of ascites with diuretics, paracentesis or peritoneovenous shunt[2], and the palliation of symptoms such as reduction of pruritus with ursodeoxycholic acid (UDCA) in cholestasis[3].

It is also useful to have markers which might predict the outcome of initial treatment in order to select those patients who may respond, as is done in chronic viral hepatitis in which virus elimination can be predicted to some extent[4]. All other changes found during treatment, i.e. in laboratory values, histological findings, imaging or pressure measurements can be classified as surrogate markers, the value of which is disputed (Table 2).

Table 1 Aims of treatment in chronic liver disorders

•	Eliminate factors causing disease (iron, copper, virus, alcohol, cholestasis (?))	
•	If impossible:	Slow down progression to cirrhosis (→ survival↑)
		Eliminate or reduce impact of complications (→ survival↑)
		Improve symptoms
		Improve 'markers'

Table 2 Markers of success in the treatment of chronic liver diseases

True success markers	• Survival • Reduction of certain events (LTX, complications) • Reduction of symptoms
Effects up to now only shown for complications (variceal bleeding, ascites) and some symptoms	
Predictive markers	• Treatment outcome (i.e. virus elimination)
Surrogate markers	• Laboratory values • Histology (?) • Quantitative liver function tests • Imaging procedures and pressure measurements

A 'good' surrogate marker should have the following characteristics[3]:

- the test should have prognostic value in the particular disease under study; and
- the test procedure should not itself be affected by the treatment under study.

These principles are demonstrated for the example of UDCA treatment in cholestasis in Table 3[3].

Table 3 Parameters of efficacy of UDCA in cholestasis[3]

	Prognostic value	*Interference with UDCA*
Transaminases	No	No
AP	±	No
Bilirubin	Yes	Yes
Bile acids	±	Yes
Biopsy	Yes	No
GEC	Yes	No
ABT	±	No

The posters presented to the symposium dealt with a wide variety of topics related to the problem of surrogate markers. For reasons of space and interest of the author, only some can be discussed in detail.

VIRAL HEPATITIS

A number of posters were related to assessment of severity and prognosis without directly using markers for treatment outcome. Some of these might, however, give some hints for possible surrogate markers in the future. In particular, leukocyte function (Baltadjev *et al.*), serum bile acids in chronic hepatitis in children (Lebensztejn *et al.*), conventional liver enzyme patterns (Popinova *et al.*; Sampelean *et al.*) and lipids and lipoproteins (Schnell-

Kretschmer *et al.*) were studied. None, however, was proven to be of practical value.

The responsiveness to interferon treatment, usually assessed by virus elimination, was studied using several approaches. While it is known that the duration of treatment and probably also the doses given are predictive of virus elimination[4,5] some new parameters were proposed, together with some not so new ones such as genotype (Wiley *et al.*; Swanson *et al.*).

In a pilot study, reactivity of T-lymphocytes to 'core peptides' prior to treatment, tested in a leukocyte adherence inhibition reaction, was found to be positively correlated with normalization of transaminases during treatment (Osna *et al.*). The interferon-alpha stimulated production of interleukin-6 (IL-6) and TNF-alpha by peripheral blood mononuclear cells (PBMC), when used in a two-dimensional analysis, was also found to be predictive for the treatment effect. The slope of the function $c(\text{IL-6}) = a \times c\ (\text{TNF})$ was significantly different between responders and non-responders (Figure 1). This finding might also be useful for better understanding of the treatment effects (Kawamura *et al.*). The idea that hepatic iron might be a predictive marker for the response to interferon in chronic hepatitis C was not confirmed in another interesting study (Swanson *et al.*).

CHOLESTASIS

Although the treatment of cholestatic liver disease has been widely studied[3,6], only a few posters were devoted to possible markers in addition to those already used, such as histology[3,6] or serum enzymes[3]. Some new parameters were proposed, such as aminopeptidase M, an enzyme degrading biologically active peptides (substance P, enkephalins, bradykinin, angiotensin) (Janas; Warnawin *et al.*) and phospholipid methyltransferase (Verma *et al.*). The latter was, however, only studied in hamsters, while the former was shown to be highly elevated in children with cholestatic disorders.

An interesting study used several standard and dynamic tests of liver function such as bilirubin, albumin, galactose elimination capacity (GEC) and bromsulphthalein (BSP) clearance coefficients to predict survival in patients with primary biliary cirrhosis (PBC) under colchicine treatment. Treatment status was the most important predictor of survival followed by bilirubin, BSP-K_1 (reflecting liver blood flow) and albumin. Hepatic excretion was most sensitively measured by BSP-K_2, followed by bilirubin; and hepatic synthetic function was better measured by GEC than by albumin or prothrombin index (Figure 2). The authors introduced the concept of 'sharp' and 'blunt' tests, where sharp tests become abnormal earlier during the course of the disease and can be better used as markers for treatment effects, and blunt tests become abnormal later and can better be used to assess prognosis. This might be a helpful concept for strategies of timing of liver transplantation. However, the blunt tests are probably better surrogate markers since they would reflect an influence of treatment on survival if a change occurred during therapy.

Treatment effects were also studied using cryoglobulins and antimitochondrial antibodies over several years in patients with PBC (Delpre *et al.*). The authors showed that cryoprecipitates disappeared and titres of AMA

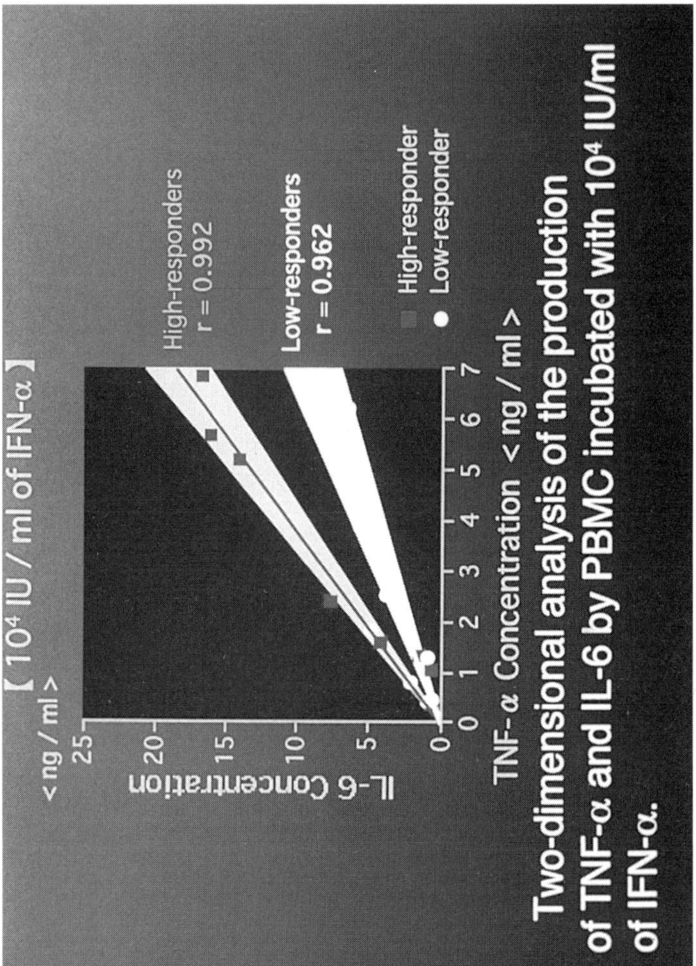

Fig. 1 Two-dimensional analysis of the production of TNF-alpha and IL-6 by PBMC incubated with 10^4 IU/ml of interferon-alpha (Kawamura *et al.*)

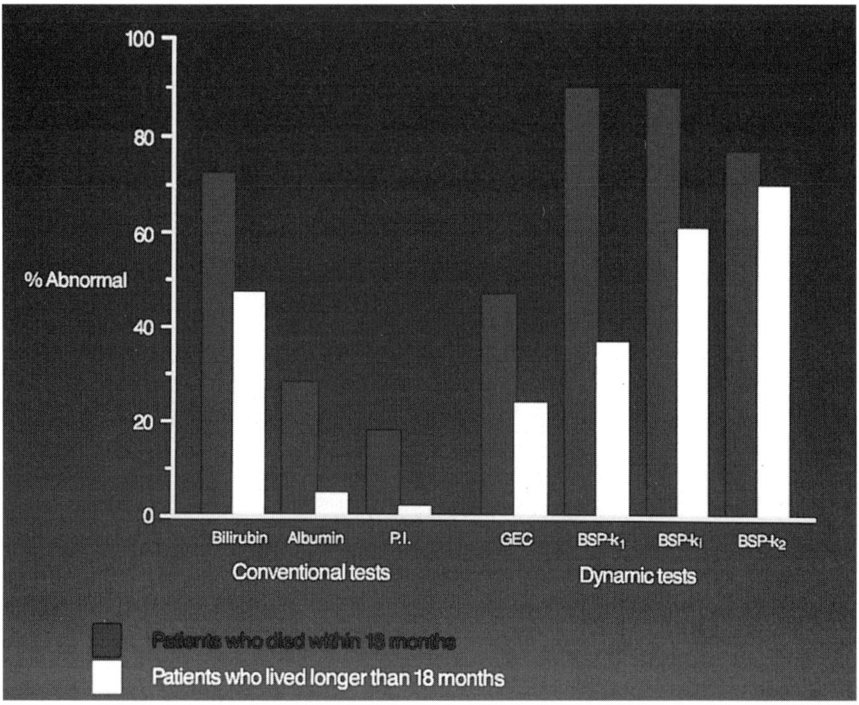

Fig. 2 Percentage of abnormal results of different conventional and dynamic liver tests in patients with chronic liver disease who died or survived during 18 months follow-up (Warnes *et al.*)

decreased, while antinuclear antibodies newly appeared after several years. Interesting studies showed that adhesion molecules, in particular soluble intercellular adhesion molecule 1 (ICAM-1), are increased in serum of patients with PBC and primary sclerosing cholangitis (PSC), compared to alcoholic liver disease and healthy controls. This increase is dependent on the stage of PBC (Figure 3) (Lim *et al.*). The authors furthermore showed that levels of ICAM-1 decreased in some patients treated with either UDCA or azathioprine and prednisone (Figure 4). There was, however, a wide overlap between groups and treatment effects were not very consistent in all patients. This finding might however be further pursued to add another parameter to the arsenal of immune parameters available. The character of ICAM-1 as a surrogate marker needs to be proven in controlled trials.

The same group provided data on the effects of UDCA treatment on the hepatic uptake and excretion of ^{75}SeHCAT, a labelled analogue of taurocholate. They showed that hepatic uptake was normal in PBC and PSC and higher when compared to patients with other forms of cirrhosis, while excretion was significantly decreased when compared to controls and other cirrhotics (Figure 5) (Jazrawi *et al.*). There was again a large overlap between groups, however. UDCA treatment for 3 months did not affect uptake consistently but increased excretion of SeHCAT in all but three of 14 patients (Figure 6). Thus, this

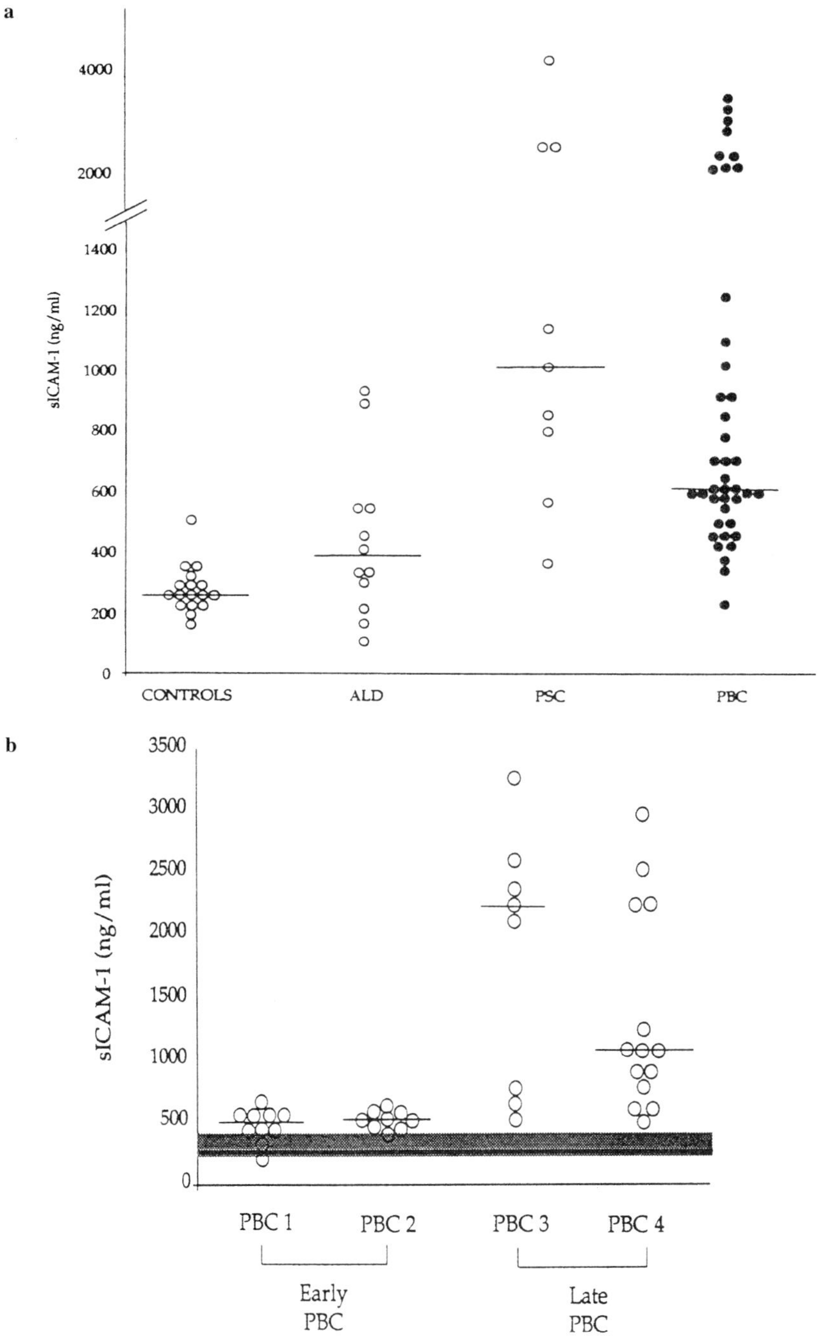

Fig. 3 (a) Serum soluble ICAM-1 levels in patients with cholestatic and alcoholic liver diseases (Lim *et al.*) (b) Serum soluble ICAM-1 levels in patients with different stages of PBC (Lim *et al.*)

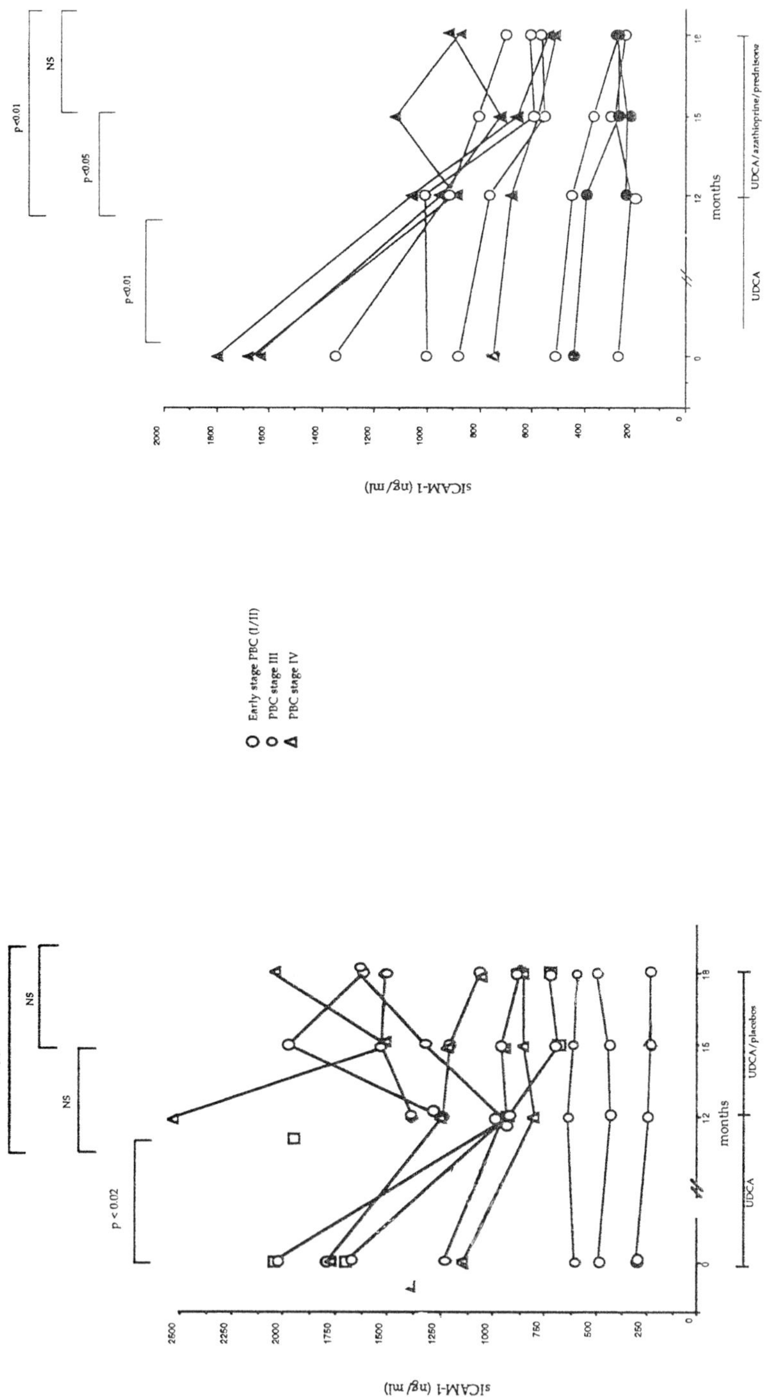

Fig. 4 Effect of UDCA treatment on soluble ICAM-1 levels in PBC (left) and of treatment with preduisone and azathioprine (right) (Lim *et al.*)

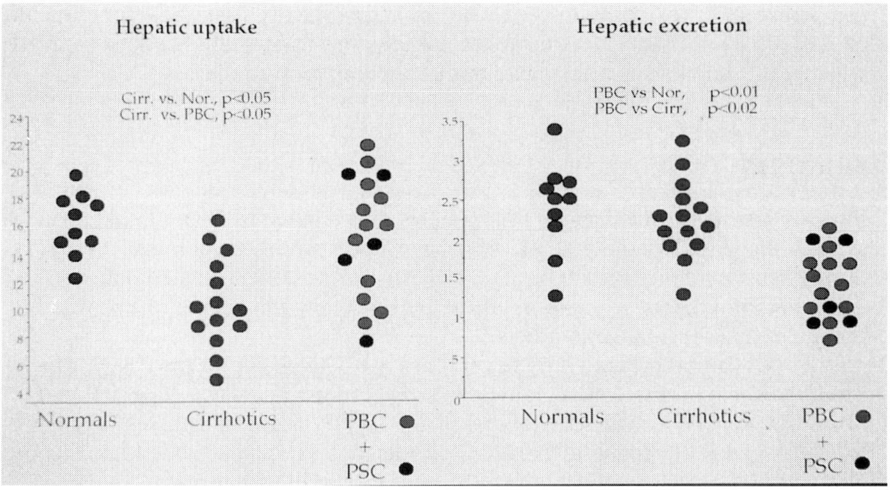

Fig. 5 Hepatic uptake and excretion as measured by SeHCAT test (Jazrawi *et al.*)

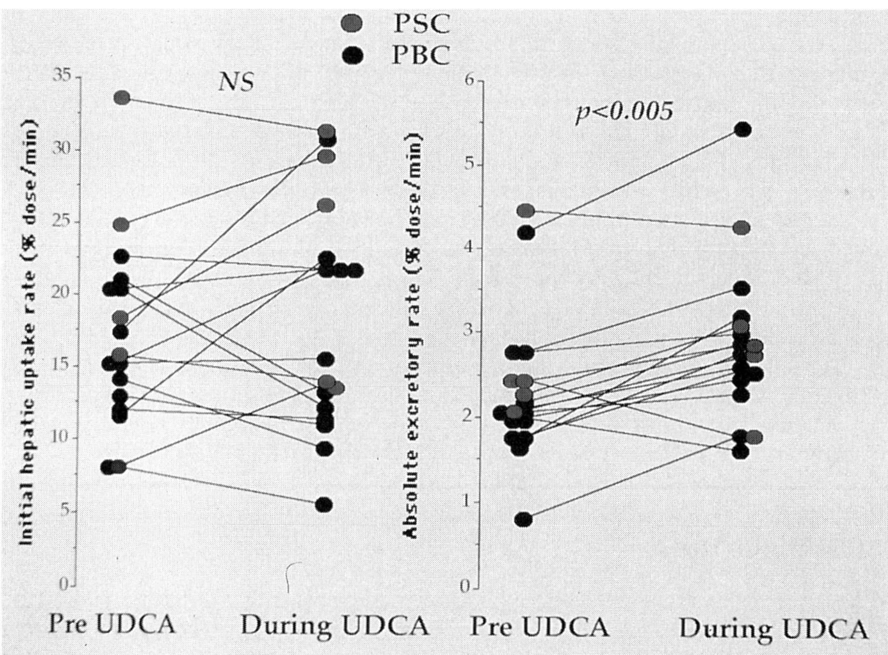

Fig. 6 Effect of UDCA treatment on hepatic uptake and excretion as measured by the SeCHCAT test (Jazrawi *et al.*)

measurement gives some information on a specifically disturbed function in cholestatic liver disease. It is however not easy to obtain and it has to be proved whether it is suitable as a surrogate marker in long term studies.

FIBROSIS

Fibrosis results from enhanced fibrogenesis over fibrolysis. Some markers such as procollagen III peptide (P III NP) have been proposed and used to assess fibrogenesis-on a day-to-day basis[7]. A number of posters presented data on this and other parameters, as markers of the presence and the degree of fibrosis, for prognosis and for treatment effects.

P III NP can be measured by several assays. The choice of the assay affects results to some extent. It was claimed that by combining assays, degradation, i.e. fibrolysis, may be measured (Smith *et al.*). P III NP measurement was suggested for the staging of alcoholic cirrhosis (Rodrigues *et al.*) and was found to be elevated in the bile of patients with PSC and PBC (Gillessen *et al.*).

In children, levels of connective tissue peptides reflect body growth more than hepatic fibrosis. By relating P III NP and procollagen IV peptide to procollagen I peptide, this can be overcome as shown nicely by Kardorf *et al.* This ratio had a very good prognostic power in children.

Another study showed that P III NP levels, as well as concentrations of hyaluronan, may be useful for assessing prognosis in patients with PBC (Remmel *et al.*).

Treatment with UDCA in PBC resulted in no change in P III NP levels but in an increase of collagen IV (C IV). The ratio C IV/ P III NP was best suited to detect favourable courses under treatment (Oesterling *et al.*). There seems to be an antifibrotic effect of UDCA. Both results have to be proven in large-scale clinical trials, since another study found somewhat different results. The combination of UDCA and colchicine even increased P III NP (Figure 7) (Goddard *et al.*).

Serum tenascin was found to reflect perisinusoidal and not portal fibrogenesis, and levels were therefore increased in chronic viral hepatitis but not in PBC. Tenascin levels declind by more than 50% at the end of and six months after interferon treatment in chronic hepatitis patients (Table 4) (Libuda *et al.*). This finding should certainly be further pursued.

A study in rats with bile duct ligation found that treatment with silimarin lowered serum P III NP as well as hydroxyproline levels in the liver in parallel, indicating an antifibrotic effect of this drug, at least in animals, and again the ability of P III NP to assess antifibrotic effects of treatment (Boigk *et al.*).

COMPLICATIONS

A variety of markers and techniques were studied regarding different complications of cirrhosis and portal hypertension. Most were, however, related to assessment of severity or prognosis and not to treatment effects.

It was found that sICAM-1 is elevated in alcoholic cirrhosis (although much less than in PBC as shown by the same group) and is related to histological

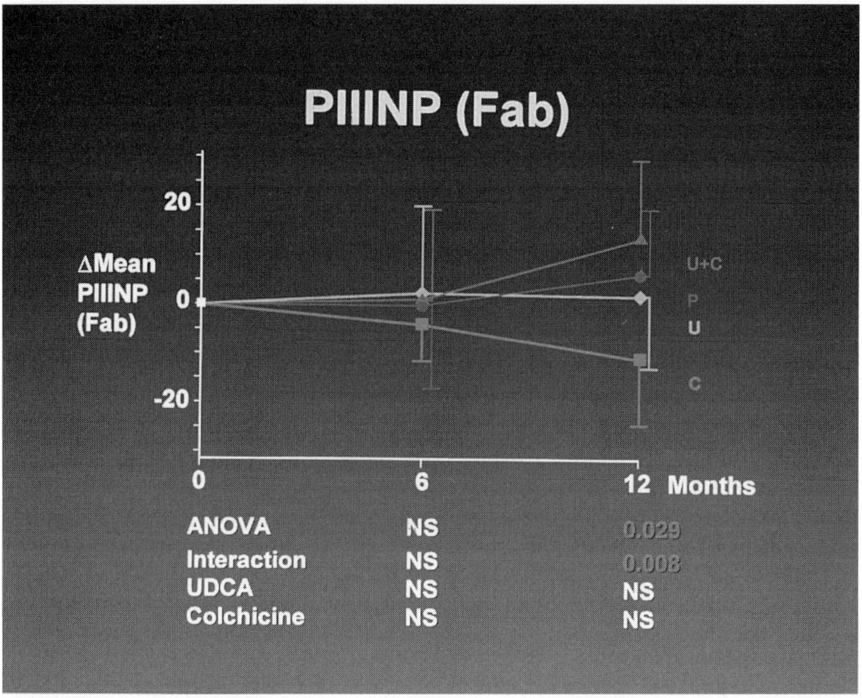

Fig. 7 Effect of treatment with UDCA or colchicine or a combination of both on P III NP levels in patients with PBC (Goddard *et al.*)

Table 4 Serum tenascin in different forms of liver disease and with interferon treatment in chronic viral hepatitis (Libuda *et al.*)

CON	*ALH-C*	*PBCI/II*	*PBCIII/IV*	*HEP*	*HEP-6*	*HEP-12*
n=22	*n*=20	*n*=11	*n*=9	*n*=12	*n*=12	*n*=12
107±32	318±104	78±26	84±29	785±169	341±124	354±112

CON, controls; ALH-C, alcoholic hepatitis/cirrhosis; HEP, chronic hepatitis B (*n*=5) and C (*n*=7) before, at the end of (HEP-6) and 6 months after (HEP-12) interferon-therapy. ALH-C/HEP/HEP-6/HEP-12 vs. CON/PBCI-IV: $p<0.01$; ALH-C/HEP-6/HEP-12 vs. HEP: $p<0.05$

severity but not to general immune activation (Douds *et al.*). Lymphocyte proliferation was compromised and the production of cytokines IL-2 and interferon gamma was increased in cirrhosis (Koch *et al.*). Alpha-fetoprotein concentration was claimed to be a marker of activity of cirrhosis and was reduced by silimarin treatment. Alpha-fetoprotein variants were not significantly different (Turecky *et al.*). The percentage of choledocholithiasis in patients with different forms of cirrhosis was higher in alcoholics and PBC and correlated with the Child classification (Stardelova *et al.*). The value of duplex sonography for the assessment of portal hypertension was stressed but no significant correlation with the degree of liver dysfunction, as tested by the Child–Pugh criteria, was found (Grigarescu *et al.*; Badea *et al.*). Subclinical encephalopathy can be assessed by computer assisted testing of basic cognitive variables. The results are correlated with the Child classification (Wein *et al.*).

Often overlooked malnutrition might be a good clinical marker for severity assessment in cirrhosis. In an interesting study it was found that prealbumin and retinol binding protein (RBP) are better than conventional parameters for assessment of malnutrition in cirrhosis. There is a good correlation with the Child–classification although the number of patients with Child C was rather small in this study (Lepczynski-Birke *et al.*). (Table 5, Figure 8).

Prognosis was assessed by clinical parameters (Vacariu *et al.*). Variceal bleeding could be predicted using indocyanine green clearance (ICG), monoethylglycine xylide formation (MEGX) and Child–Pugh score (Table 6). These findings, when confirmed, might help in selecting patients for prophylactic treatment (Beyer *et al.*).

Donor livers could be better selected by MEGX testing although the predictive value was only 63.6% (Casagrande *et al.*).

Only one study tested parameters of quality of life under treatment (Nedogoda *et al.*). Treatment was somewhat unconventional and consisted of calcium antagonists, beta blockers, angiotensin converting enzyme inhibitors and taurine. However, this study points to the necessity of including such parameters in clinical trials.

QUANTITATIVE LIVER FUNCTION TESTS AND SCORES

Since it is still unknown which particular mechanism of hepatocellular dysfunction is most important for ill health or death in liver disease, and the liver, in contrast to the kidney, has so many functions, no single liver test is as yet generally accepted as a major determinant of liver function (and probably never

Table 5 Parameters of nutrition in patients with liver cirrhosis of different severity (Lepczynski-Birke *et al.*)

		Female				*Male*			
		Liver cirrhosis			*Controls*	*Liver cirrhosis*			*Controls*
Child–Pugh		*A*	*B*	*C*		*A*	*B*	*C*	
(No.)		*(39)*	*(8)*	*(3)*	*(50)*	*(52)*	*(26)*	*(2)*	*(80)*
BMI	kg/m^2	26.5	22.9	22.3	24.4	26.8	25.5	25.8	25.3
BCM	%	32.9	34.3	31.6	36.6*	39.3	37.8	41.0	45.0*
LBM	%	67.3	73.0	69.0	71.4*	76.6	77.3	87.1	81.5*
Fat	%	32.7	27.0	31.0	28.7*	23.3	22.8	12.9	18.6*
Albumin	g/dl	4.1	3.4	3.5	4.4	4.4	4.2	2.9	4.7*
RBP	mg/dl	2.7	1.2	0.7**	4.5*	2.3	1.2	0.5**	5.4*
Prealbumin	mg/dl	16.5	6.9	6.2**	26.9*	15.0	9.3	3.3**	32.8*

*$p<0.05$ between Child A and controls; **$p<0.05$ within Child; BMI, body mass index; BCM, body cell mass; LBM, lean body mass

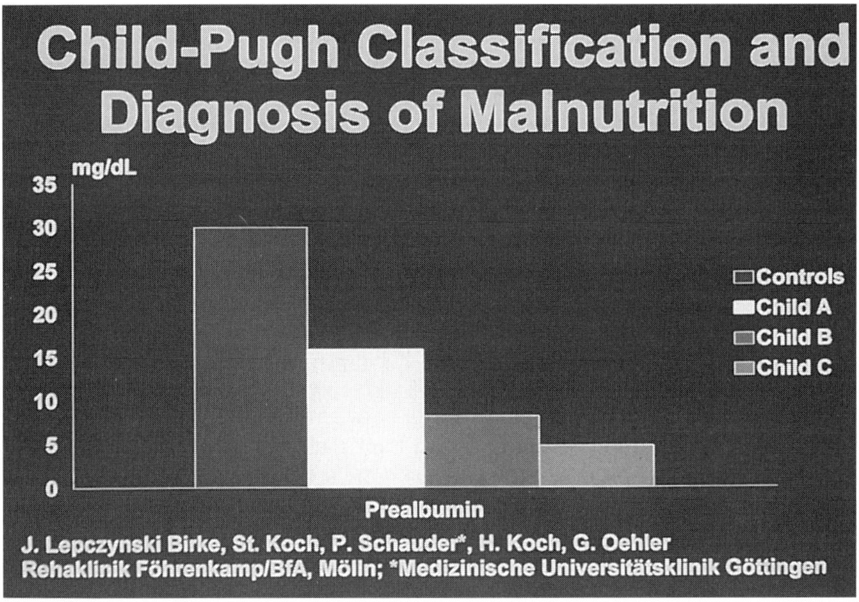

Fig. 8 Prealbumin levels in controls and patients with liver cirrhosis of different Child–Pugh classification (Lepczynski–Birke *et al.*)

Table 6 Sensitivity, specificity and positive predictive value for identification of patients at risk from variceal bleeding (Beyer *et al.*)

Variable	*Prognostic sensitivity (%)*	*Prognostic specificity (%)*	*Predictive value of positive results (%)*
Child–Pugh score	85.4	56.1	44.9
MEGX (μg/L)	88.6	70.0	56.2
ICG Rmax (%)	94.1	60.7	55.6

Cut-off values: Child–Pugh score, 8 points; ICG Rmax, 50%; MEGX, 20μg/L

will be). Scores have been developed to assess prognosis in different types of liver disease but are not widely used. Several studies investigated the role of scores and quantitative liver function tests in assessing severity and prognosis of liver disease. It was again found that the Child–Pugh classification does not predict short-term prognosis very effectively (Zaborowski *et al.*). The MEGX test correlated relatively well with Child–Pugh scores (Fabris *et al.*). The galactose elimination capacity (GEC) was different in fatty liver and cirrhosis and correlated well with several conventional liver tests (Benjoseph *et al.*) but not with the Child classification, while prealbumin and cholinesterase activity did (Kupcova *et al.*). Biotransformation of theophylline and antipyrine was most abnormal in Child C patients (Kupcova *et al.*).

SOME STUDIES AIMED AT ASSESSING TREATMENT EFFECTS

MEGX was found not to change under treatment with UDCA, interferon or silibinin, while conventional liver tests did (Virussi *et al.*). Similar findings for GEC were reported by others (Becarello *et al.*), indicating that changes in conventional liver tests are more easily achieved and probably of little importance when neither quantitative liver function tests nor other proven markers change.

A simple score based on conventional liver function tests (albumin, gamma globulins, AST, bilirubin and creatinine) was again proposed for assessing treatment and was found to correlate with the Child score but not very well with GEC (Krastev).

Using cessation of alcohol intake as a therapeutic measure, Lotterer *et al.* found GEC and aminopyrine breath test (ABT) changes over time to be very sensitive for the detection of differences between patients who did or did not stop drinking (Figure 9, Table 7). From their data they were able to calculate sample sizes necessary for clinical trials and the necessary differences in GEC to reach statistical significance in treatment trials (Table 8). Using GEC or ABT, the numbers needed to detect treatment effects will be much smaller than those using survival analysis. Very similar data were provided by Merkel *et al.* using a comparable approach. GEC was found to be correlated with the risk of death. This suggests that GEC changes over time might reasonably be used as a surrogate marker for death in drug trials in cirrhosis.

SUMMARY AND CONCLUSION

The posters presented a wide array of proposed and used markers of severity and prognosis of liver disease. There was much less data on markers fulfilling the criteria of a surrogate marker in treatment studies.

For *viral hepatitis*, markers of immune system function, such as peripheral blood mononuclear cells, might eventually be helpful, and should be further

Table 7 Quantitative liver function tests (Lotterer *et al.*)

Time point	*GEC (mg/min/kg)*	*ABT (%dose × kg/mmolCO$_2$)*	*SCI (ml/min/kg)*
Non-abstinent group			
Start	4.8 (3.3–5.8)	0.25 (0.04–0.76)	6.2 (3.9–8.8)
End	3.0* (2.1–5.2)	0.10** (0.02–0.48)	5.8 (2.8–9.0)
Abstinent group			
Start	3.0[a] (1.5–4.9)	0.16[b] (0.01–0.49)	6.0 (3.1–9.9)
End	4.0* (2.5–5.1)	0.40* (0.15–0.74)	6.1 (4.5–8.2)

Difference between the groups at the beginning: [a]$p<0.005$; [b]$p<0.01$
Difference between start and end in the same group: *$p<0.01$; **$p<0.05$

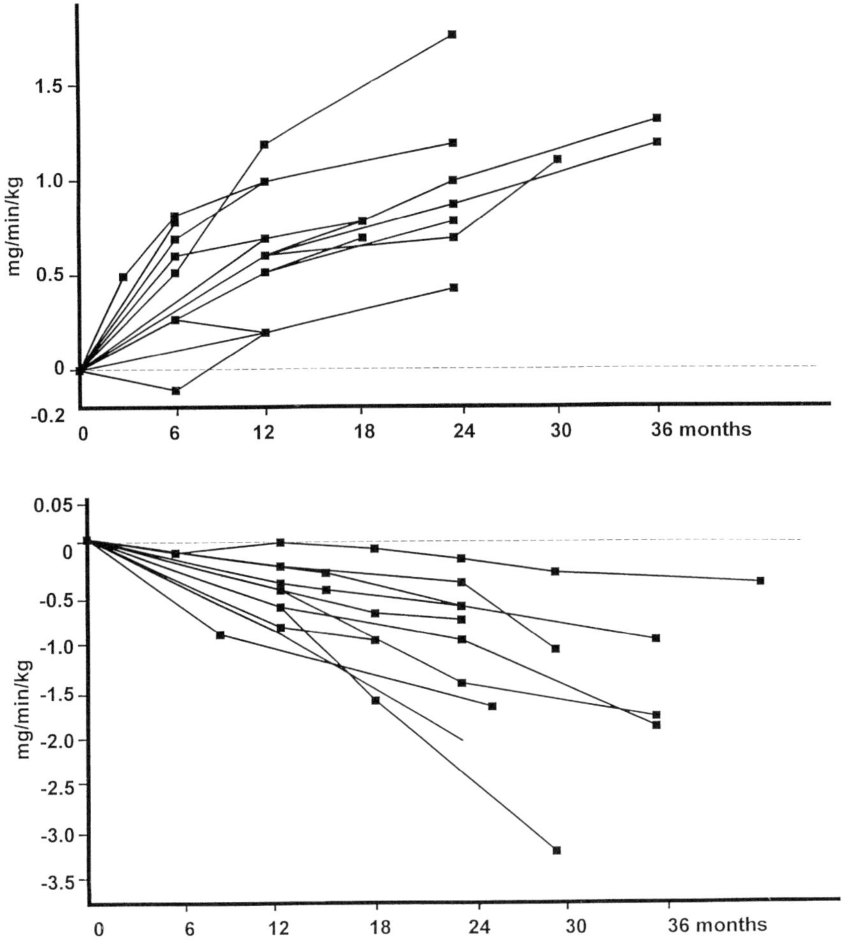

Fig. 9 Course of galactose elimination capacity (GEC) in patients with alcoholic liver disease who did (upper panel) or did not (lower panel) stop drinking (Lotterer *et al.*)

Table 8 Least treatment effects between two groups of patients as calculated by the change of galactose elimination capacity over time (Lotterer *et al.*)

Number of patients per group	*Change of GEC required (mg/min/kg)*	
	$p<0.05$	$p<0.01$
10	0.8	0.9
15	0.7	0.8
20	0.6	0.7
25	0.5	0.6
30	0.5	0.6

evaluated as predictors of virus clearance. The usefulness of iron and other markers was not convincing.

In *cholestasis* we can see better what we do by means of the SeHCAT test, and we are able to influence immune functions as seen with ICAM-1. None of these, however, seems to be really on the verge of becoming a surrogate marker for survival.

Fibrosis can be assessed by P III NP and possibly by more disease-specific markers such as tenascin. However, the prognostic value of these markers and their possible role as surrogate markers remains to be proven.

For the assessment of *complications*, some valuable information was given. In particular, liver function and extraction tests for the prediction of bleeding, markers of malnutrition and of life quality should be evaluated further.

Quantitative liver function tests are more suitable than conventional liver tests for predictions and should be routinely included in clinical trials. They might be used for trial size calculations, and seem to be the best candidates for surrogate markers, as was shown for GEC.

In conclusion, too many tests are used as surrogate markers, most of them not fulfilling the criteria of a ‘good surrogate marker’. Some do not even fulfil the criterion of being correlated with prognosis and some are too easily influenced by the treatment without effects on true markers. Quantitative liver function tests, fibrosis markers, and possibly immune markers such as PBMC functions, should be further studied and used for validation in large clinical trials of chronic liver disease.

References

1. Niederau C, Fischer R, Sonnenberg A, Stremmel W, Trampisch H J, Strohmeyer G. Survival and causes of death in noncirrhotic patients with primary hemochromatosis. N Engl J Med. 1985;313:1256–62.
2. Schoelmerich J. Strategies in the treatment of ascites. Hepatogastroenterology. 1991;38:365–70.
3. Reichen J. Pharmacologic treatment of cholestasis. Sem Liver Dis. 1993;13:302–15.
4. Poynard T, Bedossa P, Chevallier M *et al.* A comparison of three interferon alpha 2 b regimens for the long term treatment of chronic non-A non-B hepatitis. N Engl J Med. 1995;332:1457–62.
5. Chemello L, Bonetti P, Cavalletto L *et al.* Randomized trial comparing three different regimens of alpha 2 a interferon in chronic active hepatitis C. Hepatology. 1995;22:700–6.
6. Poupon R E, Poupon R, Balkau B and the UDCA-PBC study group. Ursodiol for the long term treatment of primary biliary cirrhosis. N Engl J Med. 1994;330:1342–47.
7. Schuppan D, Stolzel U, Oesterling C, Somasundaram R. Serum assays for liver fibrosis. J Hepatol. 1995;22:(Suppl 2):82–8.

Concluding remarks

J. REICHEN

The use of surrogate markers in the assessment of treatment has become an important topic in hepatology as witnessed by the excellent attendance at this meeting after a gruelling Basel Liver Week. Other specialties, for example, cardiologists and infectious disease specialists, are in advance in this issue compared to hepatologists. We were therefore particularly grateful to have their experience presented in the form of the contributions of Dr Wilson and Dr Aboulker. An important aspect of all surrogate markers is their acceptance by regulatory agencies. Unfortunately, Dr Peck was unwilling to bring his contribution to paper. Some of his thoughts can nevertheless be followed from his abstract (Chapter 3). An important lesson from his talk was that the involvement of regulatory agencies is highly desirable at the design stage of clinical studies, in particular when there are no generally accepted and validated surrogate markers for the disease under study.

The main reason for organizing this workshop is obvious: chronic liver diseases generally run a prolonged course and, therefore, hard endpoints are difficult to attain. This has become a really burning issue since different active treatments of liver disease are available. We have to concede, however, that for none of them is there unequivocal proof that they prolong life. In the case of a 'curable' disease such as viral hepatitis, this will not be absolutely mandatory since eradication of the virus is presumably a pretty good surrogate marker, as pointed out by Dr Almasio.

The situation is much more complicated when we are dealing with patients with cirrhosis. Dr McIntyre clearly demonstrated the flaws of the most often used surrogate marker in this setting, the Child classification and its variations. The Child classification has great appeal to clinicians and health care providers since it relies on easily obtained clinical and biochemical parameters and thereby does not add cost to care. However, if we are to continue to use it, it needs revalidation with respect to certain definitions, and standardization with respect to the laboratory parameters. An important issue, also addressed by Dr McIntyre, is to validate its use in serial measurements.

Many hepatologists suspect that the Child classification is not the ultimate prognostic tool. Sophisticated statistical techniques, including the time-dependent Cox model, have been brought to the community of hepatologists by different groups, foremost among them the group in Copenhagen. This issue is addressed in Dr Christensen's contribution. Extensive validation of his proposed models and the ubiquitous availability of personal computers should make this approach very appealing.

One of the first proponents of quantitative liver function tests, Dr N. Tygstrup, gave an excellent overview of this topic, reviewing the physiological meaning of such tests and which criteria should be used for their application in clinical trials. Because these tests often require sophisticated equipment and/or require too much time from the nursing staff, they have not gained widespread popularity. Also, it remains unclear whether they will be superior in assessing prognosis by scores such as the Child classification or any of the scores reviewed by Dr Christensen. However, their potential is illustrated by the threshold concept proposed by Dr Branch and by two elegant presentations by Dr Merkel and Dr Fleig, respectively, the former looking at their evolution over time, the latter demonstrating how the number of patients to be studied could be reduced by using the evolution of quantitative liver function tests. An old and time-proven surrogate marker – the liver biopsy – was expertly reviewed by Dr B. Portmann. Its use as a surrogate marker is obviously limited since a patient cannot be biopsied an indefinite number of times; moreover, sampling variability and variability of observers remains a major problem. A topic of particular interest, namely the impact of cholestasis on liver function, has been thoroughly reviewed by Dr Beuers. This topic is of interest since the use of surrogate markers is particularly germane in diseases such as primary biliary cirrhosis and primary sclerosing cholangitis. Both run a prolonged course and, particularly the latter, are often quite unpredictable, making clinical decisions and therapeutic assessments extremely difficult.

While scores, and to a certain extent, quantitative liver function tests, yield a global prognosis, there are different markers which can indicate progression or regression of different aspects of chronic liver disease. We have already mentioned markers of viral replication; other such markers could include measures of collagen production or breakdown to assess the progression of fibrosis, different measures of hepatic inflammatory activity, measures of hepatic excretory function, or different measures of portal hypertension such as variceal size, portal pressure or the presence of ascites. Their choice will depend on the question being asked and the drug investigated.

Whatever the convened upon surrogate marker in a clinical trial, one should not forget an aspect which, to the patient, is much more important than the degree of fibrosis or some laboratory parameter, namely quality of life. Dr Chwalow made a passionate plea to include such assessments into clinical trials; and Dr Fisch reviewed its application in liver transplantation, where it has been used most frequently (but not frequently enough) in hepatology. In my opinion such assessments should be included in most if not all clinical trials since they provide important additional information to drug regulatory agencies. I hope you enjoyed the meeting as much as I did. On behalf of my co-chair, Renée Poupon, and myself, let me thank all speakers for their outstanding reviews on sometimes difficult and muddled topics. We would also like to thank the participants for many helpful comments and insightful questions. A thank also goes to the presenters of posters and to Dr J. Schölmerich for a masterful review of the diverse material presented. Last but not least, Renée and I would like to thank Dr Falk for the support in arranging his meeting and his wonderful staff for the perfect organization of this workshop.

Index

Falk Symposium Series

43. Reutter W, Popper H, Arias IM, Heinrich PC, Keppler D, Landmann L, eds.: *Modulation of Liver Cell Expression.* Falk Symposium No. 43. 1987 ISBN: 0-85200-677-2*
44. Boyer JL, Bianchi L, eds.: *Liver Cirrhosis.* Falk Symposium No. 44. 1987 ISBN: 0-85200-993-3*
45. Paumgartner G, Stiehl A, Gerok W, eds.: *Bile Acids and the Liver.* Falk Symposium No. 45. 1987 ISBN: 0-85200-675-6*
46. Goebell H, Peskar BM, Malchow H, eds.: *Inflammatory Bowel Diseases – Basic Research & Clinical Implications.* Falk Symposium No. 46. 1988 ISBN: 0-7462-0067-6*
47. Bianchi L, Holt P, James OFW, Butler RN, eds.: *Aging in Liver and Gastrointestinal Tract.* Falk Symposium No. 47. 1988 ISBN: 0-7462-0066-8*
48. Heilmann C, ed.: *Calcium-Dependent Processes in the Liver.* Falk Symposium No. 48. 1988 ISBN: 0-7462-0075-7*
50. Singer MV, Goebell H, eds.: *Nerves and the Gastrointestinal Tract.* Falk Symposium No. 50. 1989 ISBN: 0-7462-0114-1
51. Bannasch P, Keppler D, Weber G, eds.: *Liver Cell Carcinoma.* Falk Symposium No. 51. 1989 ISBN: 0-7462-0111-7
52. Paumgartner G, Stiehl A, Gerok W, eds.: *Trends in Bile Acid Research.* Falk Symposium No. 52. 1989 ISBN: 0-7462-0112-5
53. Paumgartner G, Stiehl A, Barbara L, Roda E, eds.: *Strategies for the Treatment of Hepatobiliary Diseases.* Falk Symposium No. 53. 1990 ISBN: 0-7923-8903-4
54. Bianchi L, Gerok W, Maier K-P, Deinhardt F, eds.: *Infectious Diseases of the Liver.* Falk Symposium No. 54. 1990 ISBN: 0-7923-8902-6
55. Falk Symposium No. 55 not published

55B. Hadziselimovic F, Herzog B, Bürgin-Wolff A, eds.: *Inflammatory Bowel Disease and Coeliac Disease in Children.* International Falk Symposium. 1990 ISBN 0-7462-0125-7

56. Williams CN, eds.: *Trends in Inflammatory Bowel Disease Therapy.* Falk Symposium No. 56. 1990 ISBN: 0-7923-8952-2
57. Bock KW, Gerok W, Matern S, Schmid R, eds.: *Hepatic Metabolism and Disposition of Endo- and Xenobiotics.* Falk Symposium No. 57. 1991 ISBN: 0-7923-8953-0
58. Paumgartner G, Stiehl A, Gerok W, eds.: *Bile Acids as Therapeutic Agents: From Basic Science to Clinical Practice.* Falk Symposium No. 58. 1991 ISBN: 0-7923-8954-9
59. Halter F, Garner A, Tytgat GNJ, eds.: *Mechanisms of Peptic Ulcer Healing.* Falk Symposium No. 59. 1991 ISBN: 0-7923-8955-7
60. Goebell H, Ewe K, Malchow H, Koelbel Ch, eds.: *Inflammatory Bowel Diseases – Progress in Basic Research and Clinical Implications.* Falk Symposium No. 60. 1991 ISBN: 0-7923-8956-5
61. Falk Symposium No. 61 not published
62. Dowling RH, Folsch UR, Löser Ch, eds.: *Polyamines in the Gastrointestinal Tract.* Falk Symposium No. 62. 1992 ISBN: 0-7923-8976-X
63. Lentze MJ, Reichen J, eds.: *Paediatric Cholestasis: Novel Approaches to Treatment.* Falk Symposium No. 63. 1992 ISBN: 0-7923-8977-8
64. Demling L, Frühmorgen P, eds.: *Non-Neoplastic Diseases of the Anorectum.* Falk Symposium No. 64. 1992 ISBN: 0-7923-8979-4

64B. Gressner AM, Ramadori G, eds.: *Molecular and Cell Biology of Liver Fibrogenesis.* International Falk Symposium. 1992 ISBN: 0-7923-8980-8

*These titles were published under the MTP Press imprint.

65. Hadziselimovic F, Herzog B, eds.: *Inflammatory Bowel Diseases and Morbus Hirschprung*. Falk Symposium No. 65. 1992 ISBN: 0-7923-8995-6
66. Martin F, McLeod RS, Sutherland LR, Williams CN, eds.: *Trends in Inflammatory Bowel Disease Therapy*. Falk Symposium No. 66. 1993 ISBN: 0-7923-8827-5
67. Schölmerich J, Kruis W, Goebell H, Hohenberger W, Gross V, eds.: *Inflammatory Bowel Diseases – Pathophysiology as Basis of Treatment*. Falk Symposium No. 67. 1993 ISBN: 0-7923-8996-4
68. Paumgartner G, Stiehl A, Gerok W, eds.: *Bile Acids and The Hepatobiliary System: From Basic Science to Clinical Practice*. Falk Symposium No. 68. 1993 ISBN: 0-7923-8829-1
69. Schmid R, Bianchi L, Gerok W, Maier K-P, eds.: *Extrahepatic Manifestations in Liver Diseases*. Falk Symposium No. 69. 1993 ISBN: 0-7923-8821-6
70. Meyer zum Büschenfelde K-H, Hoofnagle J, Manns M, eds.: *Immunology and Liver*. Falk Symposium No. 70. 1993 ISBN: 0-7923-8830-5
71. Surrenti C, Casini A, Milani S, Pinzani M , eds.: *Fat-Storing Cells and Liver Fibrosis*. Falk Symposium No. 71. 1994 ISBN: 0-7923-8842-9
72. Rachmilewitz D, ed.: *Inflammatory Bowel Diseases – 1994*. Falk Symposium No. 72. 1994 ISBN: 0-7923-8845-3
73. Binder HJ, Cummings J, Soergel KH, eds.: *Short Chain Fatty Acids*. Falk Symposium No. 73. 1994 ISBN: 0-7923-8849-6
74. Keppler D, Jungermann K, eds.: *Transport in the Liver*. Falk Symposium No. 74. 1994 ISBN: 0-7923-8858-5

74B. Stange EF, ed.: *Chronic Inflammatory Bowel Disease*. Falk Symposium. 1995 ISBN: 0-7923-8876-3

75. van Berge Henegouwen GP, van Hoek B, De Groote J, Matern S, Stockbrügger RW, eds.: *Cholestatic Liver Diseases: New Strategies for Prevention and Treatment of Hepatobiliary and Cholestatic Liver Diseases*. Falk Symposium 75. 1994. ISBN: 0-7923-8867-4
76. Monteiro E, Tavarela Veloso F, eds.: *Inflammatory Bowel Diseases: New Insights into Mechanisms of Inflammation and Challenges in Diagnosis and Treatment*. Falk Symposium 76. 1995. ISBN 0-7923-8884-4
77. Singer MV, Ziegler R, Rohr G, eds.: *Gastrointestinal Tract and Endocrine System*. Falk Symposium 77. 1995. ISBN 0-7923-8877-1
78. Decker K, Gerok W, Andus T, Gross V, eds.: *Cytokines and the Liver*. Falk Symposium 78. 1995. ISBN 0-7923-8878-X
79. Holstege A, Schölmerich J, Hahn EG, eds.: *Portal Hypertension*. Falk Symposium 79. 1995. ISBN 0-7923-8879-8
80. Hofmann AF, Paumgartner G, Stiehl A, eds.: *Bile Acids in Gastroenterology: Basic and Clinical Aspects*. Falk Symposium 80. 1995 ISBN 0-7923-8880-1
81. Riecken EO, Stallmach A, Zeitz M, Heise W, eds.: *Malignancy and Chronic Inflammation in the Gastrointestinal Tract – New Concepts*. Falk Symposium 81. 1995 ISBN 0-7923-8889-5
82. Fleig WE, ed.: *Inflammatory Bowel Diseases: New Developments and Standards*. Falk Symposium 82. 1995 ISBN 0-7923-8890-6

82B. Paumgartner G, Beuers U, eds.: *Bile Acids in Liver Diseases*. International Falk Workshop. 1995 ISBN 0-7923-8891-7

83. Dobrilla G, Felder M, de Pretis G, eds.: *Advances in Hepatobiliary and Pancreatic Diseases: Special Clinical Topics*. Falk Symposium 83. 1995. ISBN 0-7923-8892-5

Falk Symposium Series

84. Fromm H, Leuschner U, eds.: *Bile Acids – Cholestasis – Gallstones: Advances in Basic and Clinical Bile Acid Research.* Falk Symposium 84. 1995 ISBN 0-7923-8893-3
85. Tytgat GNJ, Bartelsman JFWM, van Deventer SJH, eds.: *Inflammatory Bowel Diseases.* Falk Symposium 85. 1995 ISBN 0-7923-8894-1
86. Berg PA, Leuschner U, eds.: *Bile Acids and Immunology.* Falk Symposium 86. 1996 ISBN 0-7923-8700-7
87. Schmid R, Bianchi L, Blum HE, Gerok W, Maier KP, Stalder GA, eds.: *Acute and Chronic Liver Diseases: Molecular Biology and Clinics.* Falk Symposium 87. 1996 ISBN 0-7923-8701-5
88. Blum HE, Wu GY, Wu CH, eds.: *Molecular Diagnosis and Gene Therapy.* Falk Symposium 88. 1996 ISBN 0-7923-8702-3

88B. Poupon RE, Reichen J, eds.: *Surrogate Markers to Assess Efficacy of TReatment in Chronic Liver Diseases.* International Falk Workshop. 1996 ISBN 0-7923-8705-8

89. Reyes HB, Leuschner U, Arias IM, eds.: *Pregnancy, Sex Hormones and the Liver.* Falk Symposium 89. 1996 ISBN 0-7923-8704-X